A Cheerful Depression

M M Johns

chipmunkapublishing
the mental health publisher
empowering people with depression

All rights reserved, no part of this publication may be reproduced by any means, electronic, mechanical photocopying, documentary, film or in any other format without prior written permission of the publisher.

> Published by
> Chipmunkapublishing
> PO Box 6872
> Brentwood
> Essex CM13 1ZT
> United Kingdom

http://www.chipmunkapublishing.com

Copyright © M.M Johns 2009

Chipmunkapublishing gratefully acknowledge the support of Arts Council England.

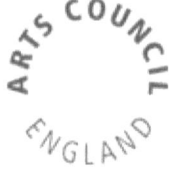

A Cheerful Depression

Whilst this is a factual account of events leading up to the diagnosis of depression and the recovery processes, the names of those involved have been changed. I will, however always be grateful for their support and understanding.

M M Johns

A Cheerful Depression

The long habit of living
indisposeth us for dying.

Sir Thomas Browne

M M Johns

A Cheerful Depression

CHAPTER 1

Hello, my name is Maurice and I am suffering from depression.

That sounds like an introduction at a meeting of Alcoholics Anonymous, doesn't it? However, if you look at the two, alcoholism and depression together, there are some similarities. It can be difficult to admit to suffering from either, as there is often a social stigma attached to both and there is definitely a lack of understanding on the part of people we know as to how some of us can fall prone to such illnesses.

I am recovering from a bout of depression which almost cost me my life. It has been two years since the first instance of this illness and I am moving steadily down the road to recovery. At least this is what I'm told. Sometimes it doesn't feel like it! I can say that I have reached the lowest point it is possible for anyone to sink into and I am now clawing my way back, gradually achieving some semblance of *"normality"*. I can reinforce this belief to myself by comparing the place I am now in to the place I was in a year ago. It has been, and continues to be, a long and arduous process. A long dark, frightening tunnel with demons lurking in the darkness waiting for a moment of weakness, the smallest breach in the mind's defenses, to pounce and inveigle their way back in to drag me back into the raging inferno of hell. Now there is a glimmer of light at the end of this tunnel, lighting the way, albeit dimly at times, pushing the demons screeching back into the shadows, but it is a light which I can work my way towards. This book is about my journey into depression, through the depression and up to the point where I now find myself.

"A cheerful depressive?" I hear you ask. How can there be

such a thing? That is a contradiction in terms, in much the same way as combining the words military and intelligent in the same sentence. Well, I know that people who do not know me well, and have been unaware that I was suffering from depression, would describe me as cheerful, easy going, laid back even. Only those who know me well can see that I was suffering from a depressive illness. Even then I tried to maintain a positive outlook when I met or talked to anyone. The public persona against the private hell which was hidden from all but a few.

In fact, that was how the concept of this book took root. I was out for a morning walk and had bumped into someone I knew. I maintained a cheerfulness I was not feeling, displaying an optimism and concealing the fact that I was ill. Afterwards, as I continued, I mocked myself, the image I tried to display to the world. The title came from that, a self deprecating view of my acting abilities. When I thought further about it I decided to write down my experiences and this is the result!

Please forgive my occasional departure from the subject to express a point of view or opinion. I recount these anecdotal stories intentionally to give you an impression of the workings of my mind. The distorted thought processes which have made this illness so very difficult to deal with. I used to joke with my key worker that he knew more about me than anyone else alive. Well, I suppose now that is certainly no longer the case.

At this point I would like to make something clear. I was not abused as a child. I am not a serial killer, or worse, I have no ax to grind against society. I have been married and am now divorced, happily, and on reasonable terms with my ex-wife. I was comfortable with who I was and what I had achieved, that is, before the depression set in. I have no claim to fame or notoriety.

A Cheerful Depression

In other words I am an ordinary, everyday kind of guy, who had an ordinary, everyday kind of job, suffering from what is rapidly becoming an everyday kind of illness.

I am getting older now and don't indulge in some of the lunatic pastimes of youth, a more sedentary life style with some small degree of comfort is more appealing. I think back to some of the pursuits, parachuting, for example, and can now, with certainty, affirm that only two things drop out of the sky – bird shit and idiots. Marathon running was something else I enjoyed into my Forties, but who willingly damages their knees and lower back in the pursuit of achievement? Now I look at my past life, and the adventures undertaken, with fond memories, and the occasional ache in a body part broken, and would recommend some whilst discouraging others.

I have spent most of my life in South Africa only returning to the UK ten years ago. I mention this because some of the events described later refer to South Africa and may have been contributory factors in the onset of this illness.

That is the thing about depression. For some reason during the process, for me anyway, the past became clearer, memories of places and people more vivid. I was able to recall events from my teenage years, some forty five years ago, with a clarity that made them feel like yesterday. Unfortunately the same was true of other memories which were not so pleasant, which were also recalled with a clarity and vividness which, at the time, were disturbing.

It is also a very lonely illness in that the overwhelming feeling is to avoid others, to shun help. In my case it was because I was ashamed of my feelings and the label of depression. Needless to say this is an unhelpful attitude to adopt, easy to fall into but hard to change. If you have tried to give up smoking you will know what I mean. It's easy to light the first cigarette, the first pack and then go on for years. However, stopping requires a tremendous amount of will power and, sometimes, aids.

I would like to think that the motivation for writing this book is altruistic, my hope being that, in small way, I may help others recognize the symptoms and seek help earlier than I did. However, there is the thought that putting my experiences down on paper will be cathartic for me, will exorcise the demons and perhaps speed the healing process. One thing is certain – I know that writing this will be hard. Not the use of vocabulary or the proper use of syntax and grammar, rather the revisiting of feelings and emotions I would dearly like to forget.

There are various aspects and degrees of depression. The illness can be brought on by any number of reasons and can incorporate many different aspects of anxiety, low self esteem, to mention but two. What follows is not a clinical description of depression, nor is there any attempt to explain the workings of the chemicals in the brain. It is merely my story and, perhaps, parts of it are your story too.

It all began one week in March 2006, the week ahead set to follow the same pattern of the many weeks before.....

CHAPTER 2

The 13h33 train pulled out of Stirling station at 13h36. I thought, as I did almost every day, how nice it would be if the train actually left at 33 minutes past the hour, and if not then, why didn't they call it the 13h36 train. I suppose then it would have left at 13h39. I commuted to Edinburgh either at 06h33 or 13h33 to work my shift in a large, four star, city centre hotel. The afternoon train had always been the more favored of the two, it was quieter and the seat next to me normally remained vacant for the whole journey. The morning train on the other hand was a commuter train and always crowded. I had never minded the crowding, except from a comfort point of view, until recently when it had become a bit more claustrophobic, especially in the tunnels. I had never been like this before and the sensation was a strange one, it was something I could not associate with myself. I dismissed it as stupidity on my part, weakness that was brought on by my selfishness at wanting space for myself.

As the train wound its way through the green and pleasant land that is the Central Belt of Scotland I assumed my normal position of gazing through the window, not seeing the passing landscape, rather planning the day ahead in my mind. Plans I knew which could so easily go astray depending on the vagaries of the guests who would be staying in the hotel that night. At least the thought of planning the administrative, everyday tasks and putting them into a time slot was some small comfort.

My duties at the hotel were neither arduous nor particularly demanding. As a Guest Services Manager it was my job to ensure that all the guests were made to feel welcome and had the best possible experience during their stay at the hotel. Of late this meant dealing with a succession of complaints. Sometimes these complaints were legitimate, of a nature where the high standards set by the hotel, and expected, were not met. On the whole these were easily rectified to the satisfaction of the guest. Occasionally, however, some issues were not as easy to deal with. For example, there are the instances when flights have been delayed at Heathrow or Gatwick meaning the guest's arrival at the hotel has made them late for a meeting, dinner or a theatre booking. To add insult to injury it was sometimes the case that their bags had been lost in transit. The result of this was inevitably that the hotel was to blame in no small measure. Such irrational behavior is carried on when it came to the weather encountered during the stay. If it proved to be inclement and restrictive to the guest's plans regarding sight seeing or other activities, then it was the onus of the hotel to provide an alternative for their enjoyment. Despite remonstrations by me and other staff members that we could not influence the national carrier's time table, or baggage handlers, nor could we converse directly with God or any other deity with regard to arranging the most favorable weather conditions, the complaints started as the guest walked through the door. As a rule of thumb, in instances such as these, their stay in the hotel generally went downhill, dropping to rock bottom faster than Paris Hilton's knickers. Guests such as these served to confirm the Australian opinion, formed during English cricket tours at the time when they lost more than won, that we are "wingeing bloody Poms".

In spite of this, and sometimes because of this, it was an enjoyable job. The challenges faced each day were always different, each requiring a different solution and approach. There were, of course, the majority of guests who were relaxed and enjoyed their stay. The odd glitch accepted as part of life, a life where nothing goes perfectly every time. They were a pleasure to talk to and arrange anything they wanted.

The staff I worked with were all very good at trying their level best to ensure that each and every guest enjoyed their

A Cheerful Depression

stay. Work, up to this point, had always been a pleasure, something to look forward to.

As the train began the slowest part of its journey I became aware of a growing ache in the center of my chest whilst at the same time it became difficult to gain a deep breath. My first thought was that I should make an appointment with my GP for a check up. Up to this point I had always enjoyed perfect health but I had heard the descriptions about heart problems and this was my first thought. I had experienced similar pain before and had not been overly concerned, they had always gone away at some point during the day. With the claustrophobia and now the pain I was convinced I was becoming a hypochondriac and did my best to put it from my mind, trying to accept the pain as normal and put up with it. This had always worked in the past, from toothache to a broken bone.

The nearer we got to Edinburgh the worse the pain and the shortness of breath became, my mind was not doing a very good job today of controlling my body! This was most definitely the worst it had ever been and it showed no signs of abating as it had in the past. The short walk from the station to the hotel did not alleviate the discomfort in the least and, once in the building I decided to confide in the Human Resources Manager. He immediately suggested that I go the hospital for a check up, phoning for a taxi to take me and staying with me as we waited. I had to admit that, secretly, I was glad that the decision had been taken from me, I was feeling distinctly unwell and in pain. By the time I arrived at the hospital I was feeling weak, breathing in short breaths and almost unable to stand. I had never before felt so ill and it was beginning to frighten me, not the consequences, rather the feeling that I was losing control of my body and my ability to control the feelings and the pain.

At the hospital I was taken into the emergency room, in a

wheelchair, much to my chagrin and embarrassment, I would have far preferred to go under my own steam. I must have seemed like a pedantic old bastard, fiercely independent and unwilling to show any outward signs of weakness. Anyway they lay me on a bed and started sticking needles in me, attaching me to all sorts of monitors and generally taking good care of me. One nursing sister told me she was going to take blood from the artery and that I could have a local anesthetic if I wanted as it tended to sting a bit, her words not mine. I think she could have been more specific! Or at the very least have told me that it would hurt me more than it hurt her. Anyway, I couldn't see how another jab could be worse than the others and declined the pain killer. Wrong decision! She pushed the needle into my wrist and I could feel it scraping around until she penetrated the artery. It was just as well that there was still the discomfort in my chest or my resolve not to show any reaction may have weakened. She took her sample and withdrew the needle, which resulted in the ruination of a perfectly good pair of trousers as the arterial blood missed the swab applied and sprayed briefly in a perfect arc from my wrist to my legs.

At this point I should explain that I appear to have developed a high tolerance for pain, how or why this happened I don't know. Also I have never been afraid of dying; rather the manner of my demise. I did not particularly want to die in this sterile, impersonal environment, and knew that it was unlikely with the care I was being given, but that is how bad I felt. My preferred manner of dying would be with a belly full of good whiskey, a cigarette and in the arms of a beautiful woman. Two of the three are not to be found in a hospital. As far as the beautiful woman goes there are plenty working in the Health Service, but I do not think they would agree to what I had in mind.

I had only been in a hospital for an illness once before. That was a couple of years prior to this when I developed a

A Cheerful Depression

Pulmonary Embolism – a blood clot on the lungs, for us laymen. That was far more uncomfortable than this episode and, I believe more life threatening. It also gave me my first trip in an ambulance. I do not remember much about that, which is a shame, as they apparently had the lights and siren going. That they remedied with Warfarin, a rat poison. Now I have, to my knowledge, never been called a rat, neither did it kill me, although the seven days in hospital did almost kill me with boredom.

The nurses and doctors completed all their tests and left me lying their on the bed, contemplating my navel, sure that everything was alright and, as I started to relax and feel better, impatient to get out of there. I dreaded being admitted, it was too far from home and I wouldn't be able to get any of my own stuff. That was an unnecessary concern, however, as, after a couple of hours I was told there was no problem with my heart and I was free to go, ensuring that I saw my GP for a follow up. I will confess to being relieved at this and more than happy to leave. I was a mess. My trouser legs were covered in blood, my shirt and jacket were creased and I looked like shit. The only thing to do was tell work that I would be taking some sick days and make my way home. The train journey home seemed to take forever. The discomfort was not as acute as it had been, but it was returning. Baffling – had they not said that there was nothing physiologically wrong with me? With that certainty I resolved to try and ignore it, feeling better when I got home and climbed into bed.

I managed to see one of the doctors the next day, not my usual doctor but one I had seen on occasion. By the time I went in to see Brenda the shortness of breath and pain in the chest had returned. Of this I was glad; you know what it's like. You go to the dentist or doctor with some ache or pain and, when you get there it's gone. Anyway, we had a chat and then she listened to my chest. Anxiety – she declared. As we had been talking my breathing had almost normalized. We talked some more and she explained that anxiety could manifest itself in this manner, as well as in many other guises. She prescribed Sertoline and told me to take time off work until I had settled down. It appeared that this anxiety could be stress related. Now as I said earlier I enjoyed my work and did not believe, at that time, that it was stressful. During the time I spent with her she asked questions, which, to me, seemed irrelevant, but which produced the verdict. I now know the term – personalizing. Through her questions and explanation I could see that I had been taking things personally. All the complaints, poor performance by staff members, things outwith my control, for which I could not reasonably be held responsible.

I did not want to tell anyone about this diagnosis. I felt it was a severe weakness, an inability to cope with my job, on my part. I convinced myself that my job would be at risk if the fact that I was suffering anxiety because of stress came out. I know now that merely exacerbated the condition. I became scared of my own shadow. I was reluctant, no, I became terrified of answering the phone or door. If it rang, I was Spider Man, without the costume, almost having to scrape myself from the ceiling. I took to staying in bed for longer periods of time. The duvet became my amour, protecting myself from the outside world. However, living by myself, this behavior posed some practical problems – food, to name but one. If I didn't go out I would starve. Even in my condition I had to eat. I didn't relish the prospect of going out for any reason, and when I had to, it was deliberately at a time when it was less likely to be busy. I was lucky that habits built over a lifetime were hard to break, insofar as personal hygiene and cleaning of my apartment went. But I used all sorts of excuses to stop going out.

As a result I was not taking any exercise and knew this to be wrong. I resolved to take walks as a first step. I needed to get out and walking did not require the planning and anxiety of going to a place where others congregated. I started to walk in the early hours of the morning at a time when all was still and fresh. These early morning walks were important to me. Not only was the exercise beneficial, the time spent walking through the quiet streets and paths permitted more thought than could be done at home. I didn't think about the people still hidden in their beds behind their curtains. I didn't think about the scenery or where I was going. I let my thoughts go wherever they wanted. The act of physical exercise seemed to lessen the guilt and regret that I had come to associate with this thinking process. Of course, they always returned, I couldn't walk around for sixteen hours a day but it became an important ritual. The other benefit of this was that I always, well, nearly always, completed my chores before going out.

Here I got lucky. I had a friend, Mary, who I had known for six years. I confided in her about what was happening and she insisted on phoning me almost on a daily basis. She would not accept a refusal when she wanted to meet for coffee or a walk on her days off. She literally dragged me out. It was murder. I hated the crowds in the shopping center or coffee shop. Remember back to the feelings on the train? Well it was worse when she took me out, to the extent that the discomfort and breathlessness returned and all I wanted to do was run from that environment. Everything and everyone had a threatening feel about them. What threat it was that I perceived is still, to this day, unknown to me, but it was a very real feeling and extremely discomfiting. Fortunately my self control prevented such an embarrassing scenario, resorting instead to a brisk walk.

As if all this was not bad enough, it increased my feelings of inadequacy. I *knew* that people were watching me, seeing what was going on in my mind. I was becoming a mind reader! I *knew* that they could see that I was not coping with being near them. I did not want to be near them. I recoiled from any closeness. I need my space. Now this in itself was not abnormal for me. I have always needed my own space and have never liked anyone infringing upon it. I think this partly explained by the fact that I was brought up in a time when a boy/man had to be macho. A display of emotions was unheard of - they were things buried deep in a compartment somewhere in the back of the brain. This was, at the time, the best way to deal with events. I have, unfortunately, seen mankind at its worst. The brutality and thoughtlessness of man towards his fellow man can be shocking at times. By the same token, I have seen mankind at its best, generosity and kindness towards complete strangers at whatever risk to themselves. That was as rewarding as the brutal side was disgusting.

So there I was – *knowing* that complete strangers could see me as the total idiot I thought I was for being so weak and defenseless against the wrongness of my own mind. Yes, defenseless, knowing there was nothing I could do to control these feeling raging through me. My mind was not responding to logic, my body was responding to my mind. The fight or flight response was always present. Flight was the only option. After all it would have been ridiculous to fight everyone I perceived as threatening. But that was another worry, what if someone inadvertently bumped against me and I lashed out, not maliciously but instinctively. That would have led to all sorts of trouble, so there was a conscious effort, a deliberate act of awareness of my surroundings at all times to concentrate on, especially when the anxiety was at its highest and the adrenalin was coursing around my body. All in all it made for a pretty scary existence, scared of my own shadow, scared of other people, scared of my reactions, scared of my lack of reactions, scared of the way my mind was working. I was alone in this scary living nightmare, for that I was grateful, there was no one at home to observe my fear, my, of time, cowering abjectness. A wimp of the highest order.

A Cheerful Depression

This battle with my mind was time consuming and I can now, in retrospect, see that there were other things going on as well. The feelings of inadequacy were eroding my self-confidence and self esteem. I had lost my self belief. I did not think I could perform tasks as well as before. I worried about everything, I worried about the planning of a trip to the supermarket, and I worried about my decision as to what time to go to bed. I worried about making a phone call.

Now I want you to picture in your minds eye a 6' 3", 220 lbs. man full of self-confidence, able to make decisions instantly, able to cope with whatever was thrown at him; now in this constant state of panic and fear. Got it? Not a pretty picture! Not that most people, as I now realize, could ever see that side me. The public persona thing again. The image of how we want others to see us.

And that was how it went for six weeks. I knew I had to get over it, easy to say, harder to do. I had to return to work, so I worked at going out, taking the anxiety attacks and dealing with them, knowing that they weren't going to hurt me physically, it was all in my mind. I made myself sit in the shopping center and watch shoppers going by, staying as long as I could, and gradually building up the amount of time I could stay. Now shopping centers are terrible places at the best of times. I'm sure most men would agree with me on that. Why do women with prams and push chairs always walk in line abreast, all talking at the same time? The Charge of the Light, and not so Light, Brigade advancing at a slow walk instead of a gallop. How do they know what the other is saying if they're talking at the same time? It seems to me that they know each other well enough to answer a question before it's asked. Then there are the kids. Packs of kids prowling through the mall, sauntering, impeding the progress of anyone wanting to go from point A to point B in the shortest possible distance. Next there are the shoppers, usually couples who just stop in their tracks, turn unexpectedly or walk straight out of shop doors into the path of passers by. They make me wonder what they're like as drivers, all of them moving at a pace which could be outmatched by a constipated snail. Often as I sat there I thought how it would be a good idea to have staggered opening times for the various groups. The young mothers could go in during the afternoon, the kids should be restricted to Sundays only, and then only after a compulsory visit to church. Anyone with walking aids could be catered for in the evening. This way someone who knew exactly what they wanted and from each store could expedite their business in the most effective, time-efficient manner. This was an amusing, if somewhat controversial and discriminatory, way to pass the time and take the mind of the anxiety attack which was coming.

The weeks passed trying to follow this self-imposed regime and I felt I was making progress. I was actually getting to the stage where I wanted to return to work. There had been regular contact with my fellow managers and they had been extremely helpful and encouraging. I had dropped the pretense about the reason for my illness to two that I trusted and who, I felt, had a right to know. I made the train journey through to Edinburgh and enjoyed a cup of coffee with them. The journey was not as bad as I had feared. Again, I suppose, I cheated myself in taking a quieter train. I justified this with the timing of the meeting. There was no need to catch a commuter train. I set a date to return to work and resolved to meet that target. Was that the correct thing to do? I don't know, is the simple answer. It appeared logical at the time. We all work to targets and deadlines and the setting of this one was the normal action.

The Sertaline had kicked in fully. The dosage of 25mg seemed to be doing the job. The anxiety attacks remained a constant, but I believed I had found a way of controlling them. It was my mind and my body and it would behave in the way I wanted – simple. I went out for hours at a time

A Cheerful Depression

during the day, sat in busy coffee shops, made calls and answered the phone. Things were returning to normality.

What of the GP during all this? Well I saw her regularly and tried to be as honest as I could about my feelings and progress. I think that maybe I was deliberately optimistic about my coping with the illness. I cannot blame her in any way for what was to happen. GPs are, even with double appointments, pushed for time and with the best will in the world are not specifically trained as psychologists or psychiatrists. I believe that macho thing kicked in, an inability to admit to a woman, even though she is a doctor, what is really troubling you, that you cannot accurately describe what you're feeling. Brenda had, however, referred me to the local university psychologist, but there would be a long wait for an appointment. I was not concerned about that, I didn't think I would need to see anyone else, but would take the appointment when it came. Two years later I'm still waiting for that appointment! I had taken my fate into my own hands, where it had always rested, confident in my own ability to control my own thoughts and reactions.

There was one problem. When I returned to work I did not feel like the same person who had started there. I felt different in an intangible way. I couldn't put my finger on it. I couldn't have described it. It wasn't just the fact that the anxiety attacks were still happening. It wasn't my ability to deal with everything that the job entailed. I just felt like a changed person. Something was missing.

CHAPTER 3

My return to work followed the same routine as before, with a touch of trepidation at the prospect – I had, after all, been off for six weeks. The 06h33 train left at 06h36 and filled rapidly. The walk into the hotel was uneventful, the usual platitudes by everyone asking after my health and saying how nice it was to see me back. Then the stacks of paperwork to sift through, hundreds, I think there was approximately 800, of e-mails to read, most of which were out of date and irrelevant. I walked around the various departments to catch up on what had been happening. No surprises there as I had been kept abreast of developments over the phone. Then it was the same routine. I was back in the swing of it in no time. In fact it hardly felt that I had been away, which was comforting in some small measure. I have never labored under the illusion that I, or anyone else, is indispensable. No matter what happens, no matter who leaves, the business always goes on.

As with any hotel anywhere in the world things happen which are to the detriment of the guests and we were no exception to that rule. Sod's Law will always prevail, but that is why I and my colleagues were there. I was, perhaps, unfortunate in that my return coincided with the weekend. The worst time for staff, in particular the restaurant and kitchen. Logic and reason is often left at home when people travel away for the weekend. It is surely logic that if breakfast ends at 10h30 then it is better to arrive earlier than that time. Not the case, I'm afraid. It should also be a logical conclusion that if two hundred guests turn up at the same time, within half an hour of each other to be fair, each wanting table sizes to accommodate their group, that there will be a short delay. In most cases this can be comprehended. However, there are the few who do not understand why they have to wait while the hundred who arrived before them are seated prior to them. When I returned I had almost forgotten about this type of

A Cheerful Depression

guest. The result was a gradual return of anxiety as they arrived at the restaurant in a never ending stream. Of course, there were systems in place to deal with this. It was not an unusual event. I had always found politeness and good humor to be the best way of handling this type of situation and endeavored to return to this way, while ignoring the anxiety gnawing at me.

As with everything, time passed and then the same issues were raised at the reception desk as hundreds of guests attempted to check out at the same time. Like sheep they made their way simultaneously to the lobby. The same people moaned about the delay, citing trains and planes that were leaving shortly. No reason or logic for these people. No thought that they should allow plenty of time to make their plane or train. Again systems were in place to deal with this and they were generally effective. It seemed to me that some people just like to complain endlessly, it gives them some form of power over those unfortunate to have to deal with them. I blame the endless succession of consumer programmes on television which glorify the right to complain about services or products. It is a shame that they never point out the correct way to register a complaint, or point out that the complaint should be legitimate.

After all this I still felt the, by now, familiar discomfort of the anxiety beginning to dissipate. A cup of coffee and all was normal. Although I had not felt anxious before, I accepted that this was now going to be the norm. Anyone would become anxious in the same situation, was how I tried to convince myself, dismissing the fact that it hadn't happened before. I had, in my opinion, handled the situations well. I took on the responsibility for the guests getting up late on my shoulders. I accepted the fact that the restaurant could only seat a limited number of guests was down to me. The fact that there were only four check out points in reception was partly my responsibility. I should have foreseen all this and actioned it before it happened.

While I accept that someone has to take the ultimate responsibility for all the actions in a business, I was assuming this mantle in respect of absolutely everything. I was putting the blame on myself for every aspect of the business, ignoring the fact that there were department heads who should be shouldering the responsibility for their own departments. In moderation this is fine; however, the blame I apportioned to myself was disproportionate. Why should I have felt that it was my fault if someone didn't turn up for work, didn't perform a task to the standards required, while under the supervision of qualified managers and supervisors from their own department. I don't believe that the company had any culpability in this; it was the way I was developing as a result of the illness. I was placing too much pressure on myself; expectations of my own performance were unrealistic. I was striving for a perfection which was impossible to achieve and it was weighing me down. I was also beginning to take adverse comments about the business as being directed at me personally. I was developing an insecurity which was going to be hard to break. A loss of self-confidence that was hard to disguise.

I knew this thinking was illogical but it remained, sitting at the front of my brain throughout the day. I accepted that this was the *new* me, I would have to live with it, there was no other choice in the matter.

Why not change jobs, I hear you ask. My reply – Why? As I've said I was happy and enjoyed my work, liked the people I worked with, most of the time anyway. I refused to admit that I found the work in any way stressful. Stress is, nowadays, an everyday part of life and I knew there were lots of people who had far more stressful jobs than I. Admitting to stress would be admitting that I was a failure, that I was weak and that I was inadequate. I don't believe that I am alone in this thought

A Cheerful Depression

process. I believe that this unwillingness or inability to be honest with oneself contributes greatly to depressive illness. In these instances denial is a greater harm than honesty. As the saying goes, the truth hurts. But we're all human and sometimes it's easier to delude oneself.

And so the rest of the year went. I often joked, only with myself, that I would miss the adrenalin kick the anxiety brought on. I was becoming so accustomed to it. One thing that never went away was the extreme dislike of confined spaces, rooms which were filled with others, others who I had to interact with. I felt restricted and self-conscious to the nth degree. I *knew* they could see my discomfort behind the facade of self-confidence. I did not feel at all like the person I was playing. An Oscar or BAFTA nomination or award would have been forthcoming had I been portraying myself on stage or screen. Again I was fully aware of what I was doing, but had over time accepted this as the norm, fighting myself every inch of the way, refusing to accept that something was going wrong with my thought process. Every day I went through the personal recriminations for what I saw as failings on my part. No amount of logic or reason prevailed. Everything was my fault. I could not see that I was doing any good. Human nature being as it is did not help, it is normal in every walk of life to only hear the bad, never the good. I suppose this is because the bad things have to be fixed while the good things remain unsaid. I always prided myself throughout my career that I complimented others when it was due, pointing out the strengths more than the weaknesses. What a pity more managers do not take up this philosophy, remembering what it was like when they were at the same level as their employees. This was always something staff brought up in discussions. They were never complimented, always criticized, but never told they had done a good job. It should be written into senior managers' contracts that they compliment someone at least once a day. I don't suppose this is at all practical as it would have to start at the very top with the higher echelons. I have worked with and known many CEOs and Company Directors who treat everyone in their employ with a great deal of respect. It is, however, their job to ensure the company works to it optimum efficiency level and occasionally this leads to a middle manager who may not be as people orientated as they would like.

This raises the question. If people had more respect and time for one another would the prevalence of depressive illness be as high as it is now? Is the solitude of modern day life in any way responsible for the rise in this type of illness? Could a different style of management detect and possibly identify a depressive illness in its early stages? This would certainly cut down on the amount of sick leave and relevant costs to employers and would prevent a serious episode and the resulting lengthy recovery process. What price have we paid as a society for the current work culture?

Of course, here I have to be careful as not everyone who suffers from a depressive illness is in work. But I would imagine that a high percentage are employed at the time. I don't suppose that, in this imperfect world, there is a perfect answer. It would be nice to think that everyone could treat each other a bit better, it doesn't cost much.

It was in August that year, whilst out for dinner with two friends, Mary and Alison, that I saw an attractive woman sitting at an adjacent table with two others. She caught my eye because she looked like I imagined Judy Geeson, would look like today. She was a very attractive actress of the sixties and seventies. I mentioned this to the others. That was a mistake. They have been trying to fix me up with a regular girl friend for years. Alison took the initiative in her inimitable fashion, taking one of my business cards, adding my mobile number and giving it to the lady in question. When they had both left to powder their noses, I went across and apologized for the intrusion into their evening. It was a

A Cheerful Depression

stammering, blushing and totally embarrassing few minutes. I promptly forgot the whole incident and it was only when, three weeks later, I answered my phone that I found I had not been dismissed outright. She introduced herself as Mirren. Imagine my surprise. We talked as strangers do, trying to find out more about each other and eventually agreed to meet for a drink on my next day off.

We met and walked to same bar/restaurant where we had first met. It wasn't too bad. After a few short moments for initial awkwardness we settled into a reasonably comfortable conversation. As it was pouring with rain I ordered a taxi to take us home. I dropped her off and left. Once home myself I was more than pleasantly surprised to find I had enjoyed the evening. There had been no flashes of anxiety. It had been good to relax. This might be explained by the fact that she did not know me, how I had been, she only knew the *"new"* me. She had appeared to have accepted me as I was, warts and all. I phoned her and we talked for an hour agreeing that we would meet again. She wanted to take me to the movies, and a cinema at the university which was showing "Miami Vice". I agreed with no small amount of trepidation. Firstly, that movie would not have been my first choice, but more importantly I have always hated and loathed cinemas. In South Africa if I had wanted to see a particular movie I would go to the drive in theater. There you can sit in the comfort of your car, spreading yourself out in the seat, plenty of leg room. Splendid isolation. You could laugh as loudly as was warranted. You could talk without fear of disturbing others. You could eat hot dogs, sweets and slurp your tub of Coke to your heart's content. I would never dream of doing that in a cinema. However, other people do not suffer from the same qualms. To sit in a confined space, in a seat that seems to have been made for anyone less than 5' 10" to be comfortable is hell. Then you are surrounded by others. You are aware of every cough and splutter from those directly behind you. More time is spent imagining the germs and disease floating through the air and into your nostrils than is spent on the movie. More so when the movie is particularly atrocious.

My aversion to the cinema is in all likelihood due to the fact that, during one excursion as a young man, some rude idiot sneezed without covering their mouth. I was unaware of the glutinous brown/green mass stuck to the collar of my jacket until we left and it was pointed out to me. An inch higher and it would have landed on my neck! Gross. I suppose all this type of thing from one's youth colors our attitudes in later life.

My normal aversion to the cinema was strongly heightened by the new found anxiety and fear. I sat through the whole performance, willing it to end. I am sure that I missed whole segments of the film as I concentrated on sitting still, calming myself. I was acutely conscious of everyone around me, their every move, and the crunch of sweet wrappers. I was sure I could even feel the breathing of the person sitting next to me. It was the longest two hours I can remember. The relief to be standing at the end and filing out was enormous. I really felt like I had been released from a torture chamber. We had a drink to pass the time as we waited on a bus. There were no taxis available for hours.

I know that when I poured my beer into a glass, there was a tremor in my hand, which was a reaction to the previous two hours. It soon passed without being observed by Mirren and I was able to relax and laugh about the movie.

Our relationship developed slowly. She had taken me by surprise when I dropped her at home after the movie – she had kissed me lightly on the lips! I think my reaction was "*Oh my word*". Not a brilliant line. However, we did progress further, that I shall leave to your imagination, but don't get too carried away, I wanted things to develop slowly. I have never been an advocate of hopping into bed on the second or third date. Better to get to know each other before progressing to that

A Cheerful Depression

stage of commitment. We even won a prize in a pub quiz. I was really beginning to like her, which is always a dangerous sign for me. I have a fear of relationships, not because of the commitment involved, but rather because I believe I will get hurt or, worse, hurt the person who I am involved with. Hell, even before I became ill, I used to have a panic attack at the sight of some woman in a wedding dress, not too handy for someone who looked after weddings in the hotel.

I wanted to see more of her. I was trying hard to take things one date at a time, be a regular guy. She was most things I liked in a person. She had a marvelous acerbic wit, she was independent and had her opinions which she stuck to. She fenced verbally with me, seeking out and, sometimes, finding weak spots, probably better described as emotive spots, in which I believed just as strongly. If only I had not been suffering from anxiety. If only I had discussed it with her. Instead I kept my feelings to myself, not just about her but, worse, about how I was feeling. The upshot of it all was that I treated her in a most atrocious manner. I started avoiding her, not taking and then not replying to her calls. I justified this to myself by the fact that most of the time I was at work and, at the time of the calls, could not take them due to pressures on my time. Then I reached the stage where it was too late. I felt I had left it too long and as much as I wanted to, I couldn't bring myself to call her. That would have meant trying to explain how I was feeling, how I wasn't coping with everyday life. She didn't deserve that treatment. I like to think that if I had been *"normal"* things may have worked out differently. My disgusting behavior in this phase of my illness has left me full of regrets, ashamed and is something I have pondered on greatly.

My opinion of myself dropped to an even lower degree. I was truly beginning to hate myself. I hated this inability to have a close friend. I hated my inability to cope with work. I hated myself for the fact that I had had many opportunities in the past and seemed to have wasted them. I hated everything about my past and every aspect of it, every decision made.

As Christmas drew closer I didn't feel any worse or any better. As I said I had accepted the anxiety, the self blame and the loss of self-confidence as normal. It was the way I had developed over the year, that was that, nothing to be done about it.

I always stayed in the hotel over the Christmas period. It was easier to be on hand for the guests who stayed for the holiday. I had gotten to know a few regulars and it was generally a good time. Beside the vagaries of the railway maintenance programme that made travel extremely difficult and tedious in the extreme. I will admit to working long hours over this period but it was a pleasant change from the day to day grind of a normal working week.

There was one thing that made me realize that all was not well. It was out of character and it made me feel even worse about myself than anything else had. I became very annoyed with two of the managers. They had called my room and woke me up over a relatively small matter. I don't know why I became annoyed and that was even more frustrating when I was thinking about it afterwards. I raised my voice at them, tried to rectify the issue while I was still annoyed and failed. There was actually nothing they, or I, could have done to make things right.

I think that for the hours after I was probably more annoyed with myself for my behavior than I was at them. I felt terrible, guilt, shame the whole nine yards. I did take each of them aside and apologized to them, but that didn't make me feel any better. It came out of the blue, one minute I was relaxing, the next moment I was flying at 30,000 feet. My mood swing would have done a Harrier Jump Jet proud.

A Cheerful Depression

I tried to justify my actions to myself by putting it down to poor sleep. I had begun sleeping for only two or three hours a night. Waking in the early hours for no reason, or so it seemed until I started thinking about it. When I woke I found that my mind was racing, thoughts jumbled and confused, apparently with no relevance on the events of the day. Sometimes there was a feeling of confusion, of not knowing where I was or what I was doing. Because I was kept busy during the day I was tired when I went to bed at night and fell asleep quickly. Again I dismissed these disturbed sleep patterns as part of the work process. I was looking forward to going home. I wanted so badly to be on my own, to be able to curl up in my own bed and not worry about having to get up at a set time. I didn't allow myself to withdraw into a quiet spot while I was at work, but I really wanted to. At the same time the anxiety grew to levels I recognized from earlier in the year. Knowing there was nothing physiologically wrong and I wasn't ill, I dismissed them, living with the discomfort, chastising myself for being an idiot.

My next shock came after work one evening when I joined some of the staff for a drink and ended up very drunk. Fortunately I am told I am a happy drunk and no trouble to anyone. It appears I had a good time, the best I had had for months. I am told I was laughing and joking like "my old self". Their words not mine. What did that mean - "my old self"? Had I changed so much that I didn't laugh and joke as much as I had? I didn't believe I had become morose or anything as drastic as that, but I now knew that something was beginning to go wrong. I just didn't know what it was; maybe a good holiday would sort things out. Pull yourself together, I told myself, and hold onto it for a couple of months until you can get away. I promptly booked my annual leave, deciding to wait until the last minute. That at least was normal for me, to book the actual holiday.

In the New Year something happened that probably delayed

the inevitable. We changed our working hours to four days of twelve hour shifts on duty, which then gave us four days off. This was a godsend. Four days when I could be by myself, not talk to anyone and recharge my batteries. It also lessened the time spent on the train as I would stay at the hotel for at least one of the nights.

And that is what I ended up doing. My days off were spent on my own. Someone calling was a nuisance, an intrusion. I didn't spend my days in bed, I got up, showered and shaved and then spent the day on the computer, reading or watching TV. Any shopping or errands that had to be completed were undertaken first thing in the morning. Any disruption to my little routine was a cause of major annoyance. I told myself that I needed this time to myself because I spent most of my working days talking, smiling and being nice to people. Besides I had always been comfortable in my own company. I wasn't withdrawing I was merely relaxing. After all, I was returning to work when I was supposed to, putting off and suppressing urges to phone in sick. These urges generally came on when I was at the station waiting for the train. I know I did try to phone once, but the person I wanted to speak to wasn't available. I went to work. I could never explain this urge not to go in, I knew that everything had been cleared off my desk prior to my starting the days off. The only things I would have to face were what had built up – no surprises. I fought these feelings, again putting myself down for feeling that way. I started to live and try to cope with this dread of going to work. I argued that it was unreasonable and irrational but no matter what I did I could not shake it off. It appeared to me that my ability to cope was disappearing leaving me helpless, prone to the mood swings and the despair which crept up on me when something didn't go right. These feelings were beginning to control my thoughts and affect me physically. I felt I could not go on like this. It was, literally, driving me to distraction. I suppose that some that some of the feelings were making me think of the worse case

A Cheerful Depression

scenario all the time. I was never relieved that it never happened in the manner which I had imagined. I always found something else on which to focus my negativity.

I would imagine that the worst part of all this was the lack of understanding as to what was happening to me. I thought, was easy for the doctor to say it was part of the illness. But how could I fix it. I could not see any answers to the questions I asked of myself. All the time the feeling that I was losing control was increasing.

Anyone with any experience of depressive illness reading this will probably say these were early warning signs. In fact you might think that someone I worked with might have picked up on this. And well they might have – if I had told anyone about my feelings. That was the problem, I wouldn't admit to myself that anything was wrong with my mind, thought process, call it what you might. I thought I was being weak, that word again, but that's what I felt, weak and losing control. Control that was most important to me, self-control.

I don't know if you know anyone who has been reduced to tears by an episode of *"Neighbors"*. Hell, it's entirely possible you don't know anyone who watches it, possibly you've never even heard of it. Anyway that's what happened to me, it surprised the hell out of me but I put it down to melancholy. The movie *"Ghost"* elicited tears when I first saw it and still brings a lump to my throat, with a build up behind the tear glands. But what the hell, cowboys cry, don't they? It was disturbing for me in that this tearfulness was becoming a more regular feature of my life. Fortunately only in private. I had no reason that I was aware of to start crying at the drop of a hat, or phrase, or TV death. Still this persisted. I even took to avoiding programs that I may have found emotive. I reined in my emotions and strengthened my stoicism. At least I thought that was what I was doing. In reality I was bottling up all but my working face. I wasn't just wearing two faces – I was becoming multi-faceted. My working face, my private face and, what I affectionately call, my pathetic face.

I saw all the things that were happening to me as my fault, weakness. It was something to be hidden from everyone, no exceptions. But it was disturbing in the extreme. The only way I could handle it was to try and go on as I had; hoping it was a phase which would work its way out of my system given time. Surely, I would ask myself, the medication was helping. I was still taking it daily. It had to be having some positive effect.

Onwards and upwards, as they say. The anxiety attacks an accepted part of every day, the sleepless nights, the crying, the dislike I had begun to feel about what I was becoming and the constant battle with my self-confidence. Day after day it went on, somehow I stayed in control. But I suppose something had to give, one thing had to tip the scales.

It was a quiet day in March when I was talking to guests from America in the lounge. My personal mobile phone rang and I moved to a quiet area to answer it. There was no number displayed and I was surprised when a female voice introduced herself as an officer with the New York Police Department. This was unexpected; there was no reason for the NYPD to be phoning me. My bewilderment must have come across in my voice as I answered.

My first thought, forgetting that I was on my personal phone, was that it must be in relation to one of the guests. That was not to be the case. She asked if I knew a Linda. I did, she was a girl friend who lived in New York. She worked as cabin crew with one of their carriers and she was on a flight to Glasgow that afternoon. We were going to meet that night and spend the time of her layover together. A fairly regular occurrence.

A Cheerful Depression

She interrupted my ramblings to say she was a family liaison officer and that she was phoning on behalf of Linda's mother. Linda had been killed in a car wreck on her way to the airport to make her flight. Her mother had wanted me to know but was too upset to make the call herself. She ended by saying, and it's stuck in my mind ever since, "I'm sorry for your loss". Strange, I remember thinking, that's what they always say on the television programmes. That was it, strange. I didn't think they'd say that in real life. At least she didn't add "Have a nice day". I told her to tell Linda's mother that I would call later and to pass on the usual condolences. It was a shock, as it always is. It takes time to sink in.

I handled it as I always had. I permitted myself to remember her. I looked at the picture I carried in my wallet. Then I had to get on with work. I'm not saying I forgot about it, it was always there. It was the lack of emotion that began to bother me. I had cried at a silly soap opera, yet I couldn't feel the same about someone close to me. The one thing I can remember clearly was the prevalent thought that it was such a waste, so pointless. I remembered Mick from about sixteen years previous who I suppose could have been described as my best friend. He had also been killed in a car wreck. I thought I was handling it all pretty well. I carried on and finished my shift going home on the train as I was due to be off for the next four days. I phoned New York the next day and spoke to Linda's parents. They promised to let me know when the funeral would be, if I could get over to attend. They were very sweet and caring. But still no emotion. I had been doing a great job at burying things again.

Well, I suppose that is what they call the trigger event. It could have been anything I've since learned, but that was it. I didn't grieve in any conventional sense. I rather remembered her as I had known her; I suppose that's enough of a tribute for anyone – to be remembered with affection and fondness, to be missed. I have, in the past felt a stronger sense of loss and grief, but this I put down to becoming inured to such feelings.

It suddenly felt like a lot of people I knew and liked were now dead, none a natural death. It's true they were, but now the feeling that it was somehow attributable to me was creeping insidiously into my very being. Utter nonsense, of course, but a tangible feeling nevertheless.

I didn't dwell too much on it over the following days. I decided not to go to the funeral. It was a long way and a lot of money for an overnight stay. I organized for flowers and left it at that. That may have been another mistake to add to the many I had already made over the previous year. They say that a funeral gives you closure. I don't know. I know that I wasn't handling things in a normal manner at that time anyway. "Normal". Now that's a strange word. I handled Linda's death as I had every other death that had preceded it. Emotions hidden and buried. Everything happened in the dark recesses of my mind. That was "normal" for me.

I thought about close friends I had known over the years and worked out that they are all dead, three in car accidents, nine from gunshot wounds and one stabbed to death. Not one natural death among them. Thirteen may be an unlucky number and may not seem to be a lot of friends, but remember they could only be described as close friends. I know a lot of people who I would only describe as acquaintances, who I would be willing to see occasionally and would be happy to chat with. It may appear that knowing me is a dangerous pastime. In three of the cases I truly believed that, if I had been there, their deaths may have been prevented, more likely I would have died with them, however, it's that *what if* thing again. I had, up to this point accepted that it had happened and that was that. My new found thinking did not permit this logic and it played on my mind, causing me to re run various scenarios in which, had I been available, would have given a

A Cheerful Depression

different outcome.

Now, I have, I suppose, been a moderately religious person. I don't go to church regularly every Sunday. I believe and I practice that belief in the comfort of my own home. I pray my rosary on occasion and I go to confession only rarely. The thought that, if Tony Blair and I went on the same day to confession then the poor priest would have to write off at least twelve hours, is somewhat amusing to me. I don't turn to God when things go wrong. I don't believe I use religion as a crutch to get through the difficult times but I do try to live within the tenets of the church. I think the reason that I don't attend church regularly is the presence of some sanctimonious attendees who put on their "Sunday Go To Meeting" suits to be seen, to reinforce their sense of self righteousness, then resort to their usual selfish, petty little lives for the remainder of the week.

I would like to think I take a mature view of religion. Some may describe it as a Jesuit view. There's God and there's us. I use the word hell a lot to describe my existence. In doing this I am using the perception, which is symbolic, a popular concept, a fiery place with pitchfork wielding demons. I really believe that true hell is a state of being bereft of God's presence.

So I didn't blame God, or any other deity for Linda's death, he wasn't driving the other car. I did light a candle for her, in an empty church during the week. This wasn't unusual, I used to regularly go and light a candle for my mother. Again I always had the church to myself and could sit and ruminate in peace and quiet, which is what the church is there for anyway.

As the days passed any thoughts of Linda and the others were pushed from the front of my mind. I didn't dwell on it, consciously at least. It was another thing that had happened and it was pushed to the room in my mind where I kept these memories.

I can remember vividly the moment when something snapped. I don't suppose that a very clinical way to describe it, it wasn't like an elastic band snapping. It was an awareness, a logical certainty which became apparent; there was no point to anything. There was nothing to look forward to, no future. I remember the suddenness of this. I had made a phone call to make arrangements for some of our staff at another hotel. I had settled the time and date of an appointment.

I had turned round and went into a pub for a beer. That was it one beer and I left to go home. Nothing dramatic there, no histrionics in the pub or street, just a quiet assurance in my own mind.

It was then that the awareness truly kicked in. No tears, no recriminations, no emotion only the certainty that there was nothing to look forward to, no future, no way out. For the first time in ages all was clear. Killing myself would solve everything. No one would miss me. I wasn't worth enough to be missed. In some perverse way it would even make their lives better.

I was going to kill myself that night. I could find no fault with the logic. It was the right thing to do. It was a strange feeling, or, lack of feeling would be more accurate. The decision was taken; I checked that I had enough pills for what I thought would be a fatal dose. The information leaflet with the Sertaline said that an overdose could affect the heart's function. I had just filled a prescription so, with the sleeping pills, I knew I had enough. Next I knew that the bladder and bowels voided on death which necessitated the purchase of some plastic to wrap myself in to minimize the mess.

Fortunately, or unfortunately, even now I don't know which, I had promised to meet Mary after work for a drink. There was,

A Cheerful Depression

obviously, something in my demeanor, my actions, which she picked up on. She quizzed me for hours until I admitted what I intended to do and what plans I had made. Still at this time it was, to me, logical, reasonable and I put it across in a matter of fact way.

She told me afterwards that this was the most scary aspect of it, the matter of fact manner with which I discussed the taking of my own life. She kept me talking, crying the whole time. She made me promise to put it off until at the very least the next morning. I promised, not really intending to keep the promise, all the while planning in my head what I was going to do. As we parted she made me promise again and also to phone Samaritans before I did anything. I promised. When I got home I sat and thought about it. What made me stop? Her crying, the thought that I would be hurting a lot of people, my religion. I cannot answer that question. I did phone the Samaritans and talked for a long time. I stayed up all night thinking about it. I didn't try to take my life that night. The morning dawned and I still did nothing. Mary phoned me early and she sounded so relieved and pleased that I answered the phone that I began to have second thoughts. It could be that things always look better in the morning. She phoned my work and told them I was sick, making me promise to see my doctor that morning.

Why did I tell her? Did I want to be stopped? Was I seeking attention? Maybe one or all of the above. If I hadn't met her I believe that I would have gone ahead with my plans. I knew that death would have been a welcome release. From what, I still haven't figured that one out yet. That night, up to that point in my life was one of the worst I've ever lived through. I was plagued by demons. I know I thought that to have gone ahead would bring sweet release.

Silly, but that was my exact thought, a sweet release. I must have picked that up in some movie or the other. I think the deciding factor that night was probably the thought of the pain that I would have inflicted on others. It hadn't been a consideration in the planning, but the talk with Mary had made me realize how much harm I might do. Possibly that was the overriding concern. I still ask myself if that could be true, after all when you kill yourself aren't your thoughts self centered and not about others? I don't have any marvelous insights into my thought process at this time despite having thought a lot about it since the event.

I did manage to see the doctor as a matter of urgency, particularly when I explained the reason for the consultation. This time it was my regular GP, Ian. He was very good, attentive, helpful and concerned. I am ashamed to say that I completely broke down in front of him as I blurted out the feelings I was experiencing. It must have really eaten into his schedule but he took as much time as we needed to help. I cannot say that I felt any better when I left the surgery. Possibly more reassured than anything, but definitely not better. The one pervading thought was to end it all. Ian had made an appointment to attend the local Mental Health clinic and to see a psychiatrist.

I had to hold on till that happened. Where, I asked myself did this fight come from. My logic, perverse or not, was something I had trusted all my life, was telling me there was no reason to go on, but here I was going home to wait for the meeting with a psychiatrist. I think I was confused, probably not the right word, but I didn't know which to turn, didn't know what I could do, couldn't tell right from wrong. If I had thought the first two nights were bad then I was in for a rude awakening. The following days and nights were about as much fun as being a passenger on the Titanic. I couldn't sleep; my mind was going off on tangents, taking me back in time, transporting me to places probably best pictured in Dante's Inferno.

A Cheerful Depression

The night terrors were vivid and frightening. I would wake up and my eyes would tell me I was in my bedroom but my mind was telling me I was in an awful place. I began to dread the night and the prospect of going to bed. I would wait until I felt I could fight sleep no longer before going to bed. I would lie down and then my mind would start working all over again. Night terrors are exactly that, dreams that terrorize. Sometimes there were people I knew, or had known, in the dreams and sometimes they were about events in my past. However, the events unfolded in the dream were far worse than the actual event had been. There were dreams when there was a malevolent, predatory, evil and unseen force chasing and threatening. Always there was the awakening to a feeling of fear, real and unimagined, a certainty that the entity was still present. It was a bit like a horror/sci-fi movie when they don't reveal the source of the evil until the end. The difference being that I have never reached the end and seen this horror. To give you an example I had, with three others, gone for a hike in the Kirstenbosch Botanical Gardens in Cape Town. We walked up a back path to climb Table Mountain and then take the cable car down again. It was an enjoyable day out. I think we were all around fifteen years old at the time. In the dream the same walk unfolded until we were near the top and then things really went bad. The unseen malevolence intruded into the dream and all hell was let loose with the others dying, we were separated and my efforts to reach the others before they were torn to pieces were in vain, I could never get close enough. That was one of the most vivid dreams. The others were, generally, not remembered in such detail. Except for the force, the evil stalking me, that was always present when I woke. I do remember one time when I remembered that the trigger for the dream had been some loud noise outside my bedroom. Quite what it was I'm not sure, but I was aware that something had triggered the dream. It was extremely disquieting having these dreams night after night. I grew to detest the television programmes shown in the early hours of the morning.

Of course the night terrors only came when I did manage to fall asleep. It is common with a depressive illness for sleep patterns to be disturbed. Hard to fall asleep and stay asleep, or too much sleep. I found it hard to fall asleep. My thoughts were jumbled and confused, racing off on opposing tangents all the time. Of course, this caused muscles to tighten and then an effort to control the mind, to relax into a state where sleep would come. Frequently it never did and the night was spent restlessly tossing and turning praying for some release from my own thought processes.

They could not distract me from my thoughts. I was slowly but surely descending into my own version of hell. I couldn't rationalize my behavior. I didn't know what was happening. I was sure I was going insane. I could find myself sitting watching television and then losing hours as I drifted off down memory lane. One time I was watching the news and I drifted back in time. Not unpleasant, the days were not as bad as the nights, for whatever reason. Anyway this time I was fifteen again and I worked through a succession of friends, mainly girls, who I had known. I could picture their faces, their mannerisms, where they lived and what we had done together. It was as clear as a moving picture. Such memories, although pleasant, were always followed by a feeling of regret. The words *"what if"* should be banished from the English language. That was what plagued me the most – *what if* I had done this, *what if* I hadn't done that. Those words became the be all and end all of my reasoning.

These excursions of my mind during the day developed into flashbacks. There were various triggers for these, sometimes I recognized it and others times they just happened. These flashbacks could be as disturbing as the night terrors. They were, however, more realistic, based on actual events. They concerned me greatly because of that. I was, on a lower level of consciousness, aware of my surroundings, but my mind was away on some other tangent, reliving an event. Control

A Cheerful Depression

was very difficult at these times. If I was lucky it happened at home and could be indulged. If outside, however, it was a completely different story. The best I could do was seek a corner, a quiet spot to wait it through. These flashbacks resulted in a tremendous battle between two parts of my brain, the weaker side trying to regain control of reality, to push the normal surroundings back to the fore and the memories to the rear. It was, to say the least, disconcerting and furthered my desire to remove myself from any situations which could trigger these thoughts. That was not easy to do. The trigger for this can be smells, sights, sounds and movements, sometimes recognized, but often only registering in the subconscious.

I completely withdrew. I resented any intrusion, even Mary's concern and her daily phone calls. Sometimes in a perverse sort of way I would look forward to them, but when they came, I had to force my self to answer the phone, to try and reassure her that I was doing fine. I believe my efforts in this regard were in vain.

The most horrible aspect of this was the knowledge that I couldn't control my own thoughts. I tried and failed every time to control my mind as it wondered off. I never knew from one moment to another where it was going to take me. I had absolutely no control over myself. That was really scary. Add to that the thoughts of suicide were an ever present, malevolent force lurking, waiting for a moment's weakness to manifest themselves. I don't know if I had more control than I thought because I never tried to kill myself again during this phase.

There must be a part of my brain that makes the optimistic chemicals that is stronger than the other parts. I would hardly call myself in those days optimistic, but something made me keep going. I would have the darkest of thoughts and take myself outside, moving to combat them. The slightest event, one of the negative thoughts would have me thinking about suicide.

It was on my mind several times a day, at no particular time. The thought teased me, played with me, how easy it would be to just lie down and it would all end. Everyday objects in the home became possible tools with which I could ease the pain. Out on walks, bridges, railway lines, cars and buses became a temptation.

I believe the reason that I didn't use any of these latter means was the consideration that a stranger could be traumatized by me using them to kill myself. I had only recently seen the results of someone committing suicide by throwing themselves off a bridge outside the hotel. The poor unfortunate landed in front of young mother and her infant. There was an inordinate amount of blood from the head wound and that alone would have been enough, but to actually witness it, I can't begin to imagine what she must have felt. I can imagine that I must have walked like an automaton, there was no thought as to what I was doing or where I was going. I was outside trying to walk away from my own mind.

Of course, we mustn't forget about the anxiety attacks. They were almost continuous. I felt this was a good thing. I had a physical discomfort upon which I could focus my mind. If you like, the discomfort was comforting. I, of course, could do no more to control them than I could my thoughts. I often wished for something to go wrong with my body that would take my mind off my predicament. That's the trouble with too much gym work and exercise, all the organs and such work well. There was nothing wrong with my body. On occasion I thought about making something go wrong but I could never work out how to do that. The thought of faking an accident, throwing myself down the stairs reeked of desperation formed out of self pity and I decided that I had had enough of self

A Cheerful Depression

pity to want to do that. Besides you have to be crazy in the head to that, and although I thought I was going that way, I didn't want to be there, not yet anyway.

I couldn't tell you what happened on a day to day basis at this time. It's all blurred together, the night terrors, the daydreams, the anxiety attacks. It was getting so that it was, at times, hard to distinguish dreams from reality. My mind was playing tricks on me every moment of every day. I do know that going out was getting harder and harder. A trip to the supermarket was becoming stuff nightmares are made of. I was conscious of fumbling things; my fingers didn't want to work in harmony. I thought my coordination was disappearing as quickly as my cohesive thoughts. I believed that everyone who saw me would notice this. As a result visits to the shop were carefully timed and my arrival at the check out even more carefully timed to ensure there was no one behind me. The normal, everyday things we take for granted and do without any conscious thought were now a mountain to be climbed. Additional challenges I knew I did not want or need.

One thing about not telling anyone about my illness was that no one ever turned around to me and told me to pull myself together or have a cup of tea and all would fine. I now know of others suffering from depression who have been told that they would get over it, after all they had friends or relatives dying from cancer, had lost loved ones and although they had been *"depressed and missed them"* they had carried on as best they could. *"Deal with it".* I'm glad no one ever used that phrase in my presence. It is soul destroying to have someone say these things to you, they probably mean well, but it is never helpful. My advice to these others is – if you don't know what to say – *Shut Up.*

Although these people mean well I have found that some of them are insensitive, possibly even to the extent of being "know it alls". I have observed also that this kind of person suffers from a sense of humor failure particularly with regard to themselves. They lack the ability to laugh at themselves, their shortcomings. I believe this ability is important. It is all very well to laugh at or make fun of others but if you can't take it in return it makes for a miserable, self opinionated and ignorant person. This kind of person tends to believe their own publicity when they look at the perfect self in the mirror. They can be a major source of annoyance and set backs in the level of mood for a person suffering from depression. It, and I am not alone in this view, is best to avoid them at all costs. It is not worth the resulting anxiety just to be polite.

I do not believe that, apart from the workplace, anyone should try and impose their personal standards, goals or aspirations on others, even if only to extent of comparing themselves to the other unfortunate. I found that that these well meaning comments were extremely disturbing, and I know that others felt the same. Although I made an effort to rationalize their comments, trying to put them into context, it was very difficult not to allow feeling of inadequacy to creep in and bring my mood down. On occasion this meant that what had been shaping up to be a reasonable day was turned into a nightmare. I can appreciate that it can be awkward for someone trying to understand what their loved one or friend is going through and they see themselves as being helpful. But, unfortunately, they are not contributing to anything but a further low mood. In my case, this made further contact with this kind of person more unlikely. I did not want to have to listen to them giving me advice that, at the time, was totally impossible to follow. It is easy for someone to talk about the future; however, when suffering from a depressive illness, it is hard to imagine a future. I think the best advice has to be, just to listen and not impose standards or make comparisons, to accept that this illness takes time to resolve itself.

Now, I have never been particularly materialistic. I enjoy my

A Cheerful Depression

small comforts but have never set myself goals, such as owning a house in the Algarve when I retire. During the course of the illness this never changed. I was too focused on my own state of mind on a day to day basis that the thought of what may happen five or ten years down the line never crossed my mind. I believe it is important to concentrate on yourself, be selfish, allow things to happen one day at a time. After all, enough time is spent dwelling on the past and what might have been, there is no point on trying to dwell on the future and what may or may not happen. The habit of seeing the worst in everything does not make the future seem very rosy anyway.

So please, if you know someone who is suffering from a depressive illness; do not try to cheer them up by discussing your plans and trying to set their standards at the same level as your own. You really can do more harm than good, merely reinforcing the individual's feeling of low self worth because they are unable to achieve to the same level. They will, at some point down the road, be able to do so, just not yet. Give them time.

This meant that everything had to planned for, not just popping out for a bar of chocolate. There was the preparation mentally going through what was to be done. There was the gathering of courage to open the door, resisting, and failing on many occasions, the urge to put it off, making up some excuse or other to delay the trip.

Life at this stage was hardly bearable. For me there was no future, only the awful present and, of course, the past which would not leave me alone. I could find no peace. I can honestly state that, if depression had been a person during World War II, it would have been kicked out the Gestapo for cruelty.

CHAPTER 4

The appointment for the psychiatrist was made quickly. I didn't know what to expect but I did know that it was something I had to do, I had to face up to the fact that I needed help, advice, I would take anything that would relieve my situation. The time leading up to the appointment was filled with a constant anxiety attack. The worst thoughts were going through my mind. It was always the worst possible case scenario. However, I resolved to take whatever came my way on the chin, after all nothing could be much worse than what I had been going through. Well, possibly having to spend eternity with my ex-wife. Now that really would be hell.

I endeavored to make myself as presentable as I could. It would have required a TV style makeover to have succeeded in looking good, I felt like crap and was sure I looked the same way. Fortunately there wasn't a long wait before he came and introduced himself. A tall dark-haired man with an obvious accent, a ready smile and a manner which, even at that early stage, inspired trust. Great, a South African, he, I thought, might have more understanding of my background and the environs in which I had been brought up and lived in. Charles showed me to an office and introduced me to Samuel, a psychiatric nurse who would be my key worker. This was disquieting as I had expected to be alone with Charles. I wasn't comfortable having two strangers listen to my ramblings. As usual, sitting there I thought it would be a waste of time. They would find nothing wrong with me. It would all be in my imagination. I tried to present as normal a picture of myself as possible. I rather fear that the image I saw myself putting forward was as transparent as Cher's shirts.

I tried to explain about my feelings, my fears, trying to remember everything and put it as well as I could. All the time I was thinking – God you sound like an idiot. You're

A Cheerful Depression

telling them things that would stretch anyone's imagination. How can they believe all this guff? Charles asked questions about my past, it was almost conversational. I suppose that, like a good interviewer, he had developed the skills of making it sound like a conversation, all the time drawing out more and more information without you realizing he is doing it.

I do remember the alarm I felt when he said, almost casually that he had thought he might have had to commit me. My mind was screaming – God the loony bin, a strait jacket. I can't take that. My instinct was to run, get the hell away from there. How I managed to sit still I will never know. The relief when he told me that, having met me, he didn't think that would be necessary was immense, a palpable wave washing over me. I remember he told a story about some South Africans who had come to work in the UK and, finding they lacked the proper tool to complete a job, had improvised. It was, he stated, an example of how we, South Africans, just got on with things, accepting that you carried on and got the job done. This was in response to my telling him how I carried on working through the anxiety attacks, thinking all would be alright, given time. He also told me how he had a friend who had dealt with guys from the South African Defense Force who had been in Angola. It was altogether a friendly and relaxed chat. I was beginning to feel better about being there.

Charles then went to talk about the medication I had been taking. He thought the dosage had been too small and said he wanted to put it up to 200mg a day. He believed that I had been a ticking time bomb for the time I had been on it, if it had been 200mg from the start, this may have been avoided, or at least possibly it would not have been as severe. This was not down to the GP, she had done what she had thought correct, but he would immediately be changing the dose, gradually building up to the 200mg. Time went very quickly, I felt better than I had for a long while. Something was happening. They believed me, they knew what was wrong and it could be fixed.

The diagnosis was made. I had depression, anxiety and post-traumatic stress disorder. I would never have thought in a million years that I had been suffering from post-traumatic stress. The thought never crossed my mind. I had heard about it, but me? That was unthinkable. What had happened to my own defense mechanisms that this could be allowed to happen. At that point I was confused. I did not want to believe it and, at the same time, I knew I had to believe it. The only way forward was to accept this and move forward under the guidance of Samuel.

It turned out that Samuel was to be my key worker. We would meet regularly, weekly, and talk things through. There were also various groups I could attend which could prove helpful. I was dubious about this, knowing my dislike for groups of people and, in particular, having others know about my condition. I still saw the whole illness thing as a stigma, something to hide from others.

So that was that. As I walked home I tried to run the interview over in my mind but found my recall to be patchy. I know I had talked, for me, a lot. I hoped that I had covered everything that had been going on in my life. Once discussed like that there seemed to be an awful lot which had been building up, both during the previous year and since March and the thoughts of suicide. I know I had let things slip very badly during the previous months. It had all built up and was contributing to my present state of mind. I had ignored things, being afraid to answer the phone had been a major contributing factor and, much like the ostrich, I had buried myself away. Now, hopefully, I told myself, there was a chance to start putting things right. I didn't see, at this stage, how long a process it would be. How could I? It wasn't like having a broken leg and then six weeks in plaster. I wish it

A Cheerful Depression

had been that simple.

I was, by that evening, in two frames of mind. I was relieved that I would be getting help and I was worried about my diagnosis. I didn't know, couldn't see what the future held in store for me. I was unsure of how I would handle this, but worse, I didn't know if I could handle this. My mind was in turmoil. It felt I had no control; I was scared of myself and what the next few weeks would bring. The only thing I could hang onto was the fact that there was now professional help available to me. I had to use it fully. At this point, though, their optimism about a full recovery felt as realistic as General Custer's belief that there would be friendly Indians waiting at the Little Big Horn.

I would love to be able to tell you that things started getting better, however, they didn't. The illusion that this, like a broken leg, would be remedied by a visit to the psychiatrist and a change in the medication regime, was all too soon dispelled. The sleepless nights, the night terrors and the anxiety levels remained unabated. It was as disappointing as it was frustrating. I had watched and endured about all the night time TV I could. Why do they always put movies on that are purportedly horror films, when all they consist of is pretty young girls running around clad only in their panties being cut up, mauled and disfigured by a variety of instruments. The remainder of the programmes are repeats of the daytime shows. I wished for a full night's sleep, uninterrupted by the nightmares. A longing to lie down and achieve that blissful state where you drift off, a time when the mind would switch itself off instead of jumping from subject to subject, racing and not permitting the relaxation required to just drop into sleep. I was sure that this would continue ad infinitum. I could see no end. The lack of sleep in itself began to take its toll. The fatigue built up and the longing for sleep became part of the day time routine.

These night terrors sometimes assumed, in retrospect, amusing aspects.

There was the time I came to inside my wardrobe. My suits, shirts, everything was lying on the floor. Each item had been removed from the hanger. What a mess. It took time to realize where I was – I could see the familiar curtains, my bed, my room. However, my mind had me in a small, dark room with threatening shadowy figures lurking in the corners. Eventually I came out of it and started to repack the wardrobe, but what a figure I must cut, had anyone seen me. Standing in my wardrobe, dressed in only shorts, cowering against the back wall. I do know that I was covered in sweat, rivulets were running down my face and chest. My hair was soaked, the back of my neck growing colder as I became more aware.

On another occasion I woke to the sound of crashing. I had swung my arm to ward off something in my dreams and cleared the bedside table of all its contents, lamp, clock, fortunately unbroken. The bed was in complete disarray. I had somehow managed to strip off the bottom sheet, the pillows were at the other side of the room. I do not remember the dream, but it was certainly terrifying. It was always the same, to varying degrees. At the time of waking the terrors were real. They were in fact, a dark coat hanging on the back of the door, a wind blowing outside. I don't know what triggered them or where the contents came from. I'm led to believe that possibly some primeval fears that lurk within us all can surface in this way. I know, for instance, that I am absolutely petrified at the thought and sight of snakes. They give me the shivers if I see one in a magazine and accidentally touch it when turning the page. I know that one night I thought there was one in my bed when I woke. I got up and stripped the bed, turning the mattress and remaking it before I would again climb in. Irrational, I know, I am sure many others have experienced the same thing. It was just that, at this time, it all took on dimensions disproportionate to previous *"normal"*

A Cheerful Depression

nightmares.

The first week following my interview was bad, nothing changed. The medication was being increased in small amounts and was thus taking effect very slowly. I discussed this with Samuel at our first meeting. I could see nothing positive about the week, nothing good about myself. I still blamed myself for getting into this mess. Everything I said he tried to put a positive spin on it. It was a positive that I had turned up for this the first meeting, he told me. It was positive that I had kept my personal hygiene at an acceptable level. Whilst I agreed with him, in my mind I doubted everything he said. It was extremely difficult to feel as positive as he was making things out to be. I found it hard to concentrate on what he was saying. My mind kept shifting, twisting and turning of its own accord. I had noticed it at home but had paid it no heed. I ended up worrying about this lack of concentration more than what was being said. It hadn't seemed important before, concentration on a TV programme or book was normal. I will confess to reading and re-reading whole chapters of novels as I couldn't remember having read them the first time, or I couldn't remember the content. It felt as if more things were piled on me which I did not have the ability to cope with. Was this inability to concentrate a further sign that I was losing my mind, or control over it? Something else to worry about. To become anxious about. I felt really down those nights, with the resulting bad thoughts about ending it all coming to the fore. What had I done to deserve this, was prevalent, intruding into the performance of the simplest of tasks. This inability to concentrate was, of course, directly related to the mix of thoughts as the mind jumped randomly from one topic to another.

Through this I tried to occupy myself and keep my mind active with computer games which required some level of concentration. It was inevitably very frustrating and difficult. The simplest of games such as Solitaire, took far longer and with a lower success rate than I knew myself to capable of, I grew to hate them, but persevered. After all, I had to keep my brain working in some manner. I suppose that, even at this early stage, I was challenging the negativity in some small way, without really appreciating what I was doing. It was to be a long time before I was given the correct tools and understanding to be more effective.

I was also seeing the worst case scenario in everything I had to do. For example, if I phoned someone and it went to voice mail and they didn't reply, it was because they didn't want to speak to me. Had I done something horrendously wrong? If the phone rang it could only be bad news. Of course it never was but the feeling that it could only be bad was overriding all sense of logic. Answering the phone or the door became an evil that had to done, or avoided if at all possible. The phone was easier if there was a caller ID, but even then it was a major effort.

There was no conflict with these emotions, just one certainty – fear, fear and confusion. There was no logical or reasonable pattern. My mind was a jumbled, mixed up mess. Random thoughts were dictating my life, controlling how I did things. But definitely the worst emotion was the raw, unmitigated and constant fear. Fear of a specific can be controlled, channeled. Fear of an intangible, unseen and unknown *concept or feeling* is harder to deal with; you cannot fight an insidious, creeping thought.

And that was my life. This is what I had to get used to, I often thought. I had to accept it, I could, after all, see no way to fight it, no way to control it. I had become a wreck.

One thing I was sure of – that if Samuel's perpetual optimism and talk of an end to this hell continued – he was going to be a serious pain the arse! I mean, how could a person sit there facing this miserable shell of a man and be optimistic. How

A Cheerful Depression

could he talk to me of positives in my life when, as far as I could see, there were none? Secretly, as I watched him over the coming months, I longed for the ability to relax, to slouch in a chair and talk to him. To not be concerned about my tenseness, my body language which betrayed my thoughts.

Samuel was rapidly becoming my contact with the world outside my apartment. Mary did try to get me out as much as possible but I was becoming more and more withdrawn, more obtuse in my conversations with her. I loathed anyone seeing me in this condition. There I was mind reading again, assuming that all and sundry could see what was wrong with me. I tried to rationalize this by thinking that no one cared what happened to me anyway. Another wrong thought, but one I was convinced was still relevant. I was worthless, I had nothing to offer, I was a burden. My rationale to being a burden was to tell myself that it was pride which prevented me from relying or placing my trust in others. I could either live with this or deal with it on my own.

As you have probably by now guessed I am a stubborn, old fool. If my neck grew any stiffer I would have trouble tying my shoe laces. The obvious solution to this was to only wear slip on shoes!

If you compare this illness and the treatment to a war then it comes down to winning skirmishes, the rare big battle, but an ongoing forward movement. There have to be defeats, withdrawals, time to regroup. The goal, however, has to remain constant. It was to take a long time for me to accept this, my skirmishes assumed the proportions of a major battle, and the subsequent defeats were soul destroying, spinning me out of control in a vicious downward spiral. Strategies I was trying to employ on my own were failing. I had to hope that Samuel would come up with new techniques and tactics which I could use to outflank and defeat this most bitter enemy.

And so my life, no, my existence, I lived only in the sense that I breathed and my heart beat continued. The nights were filled with heart pounding, gut wrenching, adrenalin fueled terror. My days were filled with fatigue, anxiety which tautened the muscles continually, increasing the tiredness and producing headaches, the muscles in the neck constricting. Fear was crippling me. Fear of having to talk to anyone, fear of having to make a decision or leave the safety of my apartment. My duvet was my only protection.

Guilt and self-loathing about my condition prevailed. I was aware of everything I was doing, or not doing, and although I knew it to be wrong, was powerless to alter my behavior. A malignant force was inveigling itself remorselessly into my mind, driving it downward in an ever increasing spiral. Driving it, to what I felt, was the limits of sanity. An invidious, unstoppable force which trying to stop made me appreciate the efforts of King Canute in trying to halt the incoming tide.

As if all of the above was not bad enough, I would find myself crying at the slightest thing.

I do not mean that the tears were welling up and rolling down my cheeks. I mean sobbing, heart-breaking, shoulder-shaking sobbing. There were times when this was triggered by a song, long forgotten, on the radio, a passage in a book or sometimes a memory. I like Country and Western music, and it may be said that this genre of music is enough to drive anyone to tears. Most of the songs are about lost love. Lyrics such as "my horse just died and my woman left, now I've nowhere to hang my saddle." But it wasn't so much about the lyrics as the buried memories they revived. Most of the memories were fond ones which followed a cycle of deteriorating into not so fond ones. Generally the regret followed at some stage. The *"what if"* question invariably came to mind. Now all these memories are the same as everyone has, the difference in my

A Cheerful Depression

state was that they assumed a significance totally out of proportion to what they represented. They were, after all, memories of normal part of growing up, growing older. At this time I thought how nice it would not be in possession of any memories. However, memories are what make us what we are, what would life be like with them?

There was one instance when the mention of a racecourse on the morning news triggered a stream of memories from my youth. I sat and remembered every detail from the time of knowing someone who lived next to a racecourse through the next six years. This process took the whole morning and when I became aware of the time again it was noon – I had *lost* four hours. The memories were pleasant to begin with then the bad side of my mind took over and then alternative scenarios were pushed to the front of my mind to replace the existing thoughts. At the end of what should have been a pleasurable experience it was, instead, a waking nightmare. This type of state was a common occurrence during this period and was extremely disturbing. I had never before experienced a nightmare as part of a day dream, but they can be every bit as bad as the night terrors. It is also hard to differentiate between the imagination and reality, something that has continued, although not on the same scale, thankfully.

I have come to accept that feeling sorrow is natural for all of us, that the occasional tear is normal. Admittedly it took a long time for me to realize this, accept it. I have discussed the fact that, over the last ten years of so, I have made a conscious effort to permit my feeling to rise to the surface. I had felt that this was one way in which I could, perhaps, become a better person. I have talked this through with Samuel. Could this lowering of my defenses have contributed to my illness? I had been chipping away at the solid brick wall at the back of my mind for years. It was entirely possible that the wave of repressed emotions had overtaken me. You have to remember that, at this stage, I knew nothing of the levels of Seratonin in the brain and how it functioned. It all came down to my raw emotions. I saw this as the sole reason for my condition. Unfortunately, now that I had released them I could not push or prod them back behind the wall and rebuild it.

Up to this point I had never understood how anyone could take his or her own life. Nothing in our upbringing, no amount of books read, nothing on television, can prepare someone for the despair and helplessness that depression visits upon one. Life experiences whether good or bad, which are a part of development and learning, do not, in any way, contribute to one's ability to handle this situation. I know that I could never have even imagined the kind of hell I was now living in.

The levels of medication gradually increased over four weeks to the maximum 200mg dosage. I continued to see Samuel. And I continued to feel bad. I had managed to speak to my boss. He had phoned and suggested a meeting. Needless to say, while I agreed, my anxiety levels went through the roof. The meeting was to be later on the same day which was great as the anxiety would only be for the few hours prior to the meeting.

The negative thoughts about what he was going to say, tell me almost drove to canceling. The overwhelming conviction that it was bound to be bad news distracted any logic. The wait was interminable, rarely has an afternoon passed so slowly. It I was actually a relief to get up from my chair and leave my apartment. As usual, I tried to hide the way I was feeling when I did meet with him. To be honest I don't think I did very well in this regard.

It was a relaxed chat. He appeared to be genuinely concerned about my health. I did manage to blurt out, stammering and stuttering, some of the things that were wrong with me. Thankfully he accepted what I said and didn't push me in the

A Cheerful Depression

least. He brought me up to date on what was happening at the hotel, who had left, who had arrived and plans that were being made. He also suggested that I utilize the health club facilities in the Stirling hotel of the same group. I had been reluctant to make any overtures in that regard and he then took me up to the hotel. I knew the General Manager there and we had a brief chat while I filled in the paperwork.

Membership was now mine. I was aware that not only would the exercise be greatly beneficial in a physical sense, but more importantly it might increase my self esteem. It was also handy in that it opened at 06h30 and I could follow my routine of early rises, going to the gym and be home by 09h00.

Gym work to me has always been an enjoyable experience. I like the hard physical effort of pushing the body. The goals that I set myself have always been high but it gives a fantastic sense of achievement to attain, to feel and see the body shape changing as muscles become firmer and regain their definition. I know it has been said that the release of endorphins through exercise can be addictive and lead to over exertion. Being older and, although some may disagree, wiser, this was never one of my problems. I set myself some targets and knew what I had to do to achieve them.

I do not wish to appear derogatory about some of the other members, in fact nothing is further from my mind, but it was comforting to see that others had a similar body shape to mine. It can be off putting if you are surrounded by muscular, slim, aerobic people who have the cardio vascular fitness of a professional athlete. A new purpose, dimension had been added to my existence. I felt better going to the gym every day. I began to feel more alert. While I was exercising, I was concentrating on myself, the levels to which I could push myself. There was no room for doubts, no time for recriminations or self loathing. As I began to notice the benefits of the hard work I felt I was regaining some control over myself. I could feel a vestige of self esteem returning. At home I was still prone to the anxiety and fears. The nights were getting better, the exercise was tiring me out physically, the muscles were demanding more quality rest and were beginning to get it. Gym work also has the benefit of being a solitary pastime. It is not a requirement that you converse with anyone else, it is better to use your oxygen for the effort.

This sense of well being developed and I felt that I should start considering a return to work. I had been off for eight weeks and, with the previous year's absence, was in danger of going from full pay to Statutory Sick Pay. I could not afford this and set myself a date to restart.

Samuel was a bit dubious about this. It could be a false optimism regarding my recovery. The date of returning dictated not by my well being, rather by necessity.

I did harbor the same doubts. I knew I was not myself. My resolve weakened periodically, I was still feeling anxious a lot of time. I reasoned, however, that to return to work would be beneficial. I would have control over myself again.

I did not consider myself to be suffering from an illness at this point, despite remonstrations form Samuel to the contrary. I couldn't see, hear or feel anything wrong me. How could I, therefore, be ill? I felt a fraud, taking time off work. I was concerned about the effect that my prolonged absence was having on my colleagues. Someone would have to take up my work load on top of their own. I tried to push my anxiety about my decision to the back of my mind. I tried to ignore all the other feelings which were still prevalent. I thought that a return to work would make me feel better about myself. I could not see the harm that would result. I met with Michael again and set a date. I would return for only one day, have four days off and then start as normal. It was suggested that

A Cheerful Depression

the return would be gradual; responsibilities increasing as normal service was resumed. There was a nagging disquiet which I tried to quell, but which persisted. I refused to weaken in my resolve. I had made the decision and that was all there was to it. That stubborn, prideful streak rearing its ugly head again.

I don't know if the two weeks following this decision were any better than previously. I kept my resolve at the forefront of my mind as much as possible. It had developed into something that absolutely had to be done, in the same way as it had been necessary to force myself to go to the shop, shopping center or for a walk. In truth, I did not feel in the least bit confident about my abilities. I did not know, indeed I was afraid of my reaction when I was work. What about my crying? The fumbling? Would I be able to carry off the act, the public persona I had so carefully developed? I was not at all comfortable with the idea, but it had to be done, that is what I kept telling myself. It had to be done, no matter how unpleasant. I had to deal with it; I had to find something inside me, some strength to get through this. It couldn't be any worse than sitting at home all day, could it?

I continued attending the gym on a daily basis. It felt good. I was at the stage where muscle definition and strength were picking up. The exercises were becoming more strenuous and testing. The endorphins were in full flow, coursing around my body for an hour and a half each day. The only drawback was that the dread, the anxiety was an omnipotent force trying to drag me back, screaming, to where I had been. I made every effort to disguise this, even from myself. I refused to admit that I was, if not fully recovered, at least, well down the road. I had the medication and surely this would take over, controlling the symptoms, suppressing the anxiety, permitting this return to normality which I had craved for so long. The time I had been off work felt far longer than it had been. I could look back and be unable to account for whole days. The initial days and weeks had melted, solidifying in the lava of the mind. One good thing when I thought this was that I had not exploded, erupted. I had endured a quiet depression, one that had remained fermenting and bubbling well below the surface.

A week before starting I traveled through to Edinburgh. The train journey was not as bad as the last one had been. It was bad enough, but nothing I couldn't handle. I put the trepidation I felt prior to walking into the hotel down to nerves; natural after the length of time I had been absent. I mustered my thoughts, focused on what I would be doing, literally pulled back my shoulders and went in.

I did not experience the sense of pleasure I had anticipated at this, my return. I might have set my expectations too high. It was terrible, I felt scared. Much the same as the first day at the "big" school. There was no logical reason for this. I knew what my job required of me. Nothing had changed in the time I had been away. It was me! I was still a different person to the one of even a few months ago. I lacked the old self-confidence. I was looking at everyone I met, *"knowing"* they could see the weakness in me, could see through the facade.

I was extremely self-conscious, I was aware of every movement I made, trying to control my body language. All the while there was the pain in my chest and shortness of breath associated with high anxiety levels. I was frustrated. I wanted; I needed the old me back again. Was this idea of going back to work the answer I had hoped it would be?

Over coffee Graham and I talked about what had been happening, what the future plans were and how I fitted into them. We were to be undertaking a deep clean of all the bedrooms and it was suggested that I work with the Housekeeper to assist in the checking and forward movement of this project. I was happy to do that. It was a reprieve from

A Cheerful Depression

my normal duties. I would be able to spend time in the bedrooms as opposed to the public areas. This should allow me plenty of time to adjust and reacclimatize myself. During the time it took to have our discussion there had been the distraction of several staff members coming across to say hello. The initial panic when approached was easily controlled, a good sign, I told myself. Sitting back down afterwards I consciously controlled my body language, making a concerted effort to appear relaxed and confident.

There was to be no lingering on my part after the meeting finished. I wanted to escape. I needed to achieve the relative anonymity of the street. The crowds were no longer a threat. They were a place to hide. And there were plenty of tourists around to hide amongst.

Edinburgh is a tourist city. It has the architecture and history to attract tourists from all around the world. They contribute greatly to the local economy and keep people like me in jobs. As an ordinary local on the street, however, it's a different story. They are a right royal pain in the backside. Add to the incessant noise of traffic, buses and delivery trucks spewing out toxic fumes, the incomprehensible chatter of a multitude of tongues and you have chaotic assault on the senses. There are groups of young students gathered around their teachers, completely blocking the sidewalk, outwardly demonstrating an interest, awe and wonder at the sights, while covertly groping each other. I can only assume that the boys and girls are segregated in their living accommodation, that they have no other recourse but to fondle each other in public. Then there are the visitors from the Far East, with their cameras clicking as they try to capture every possible aspect of Scottish life. The memory capacity on their computers must be astronomical to hold all the images they capture. Men in kilts with bagpipes must surely earn a fortune posing with the wives, husbands and various others of the group. These bagpipe players should form a union of sorts. There is one on almost every corner, each playing a different tune. The result is a cacophony of sound that does not stir the blood. Rather it makes the blood freeze in the veins. In the midst of all this are the local workers and business people, rushing to get to or from work, to appointments, weaving around the groups, darting in and out as they hurry along the sidewalk. As comical as Puffins, striding along, briefcase in one hand, the other holding a mobile phone pressed to ear, trying to hear and shouting a reply. There is no such thing as confidences in business when walking along a busy street. Anyone in a ten foot radius can hear exactly what you're talking about. It would be terrible, amusing, but terrible, if one of these conversations was to a lover and an acquaintance, or worse, a partner, was walking in close proximity.

Then, for the commuter, hell on wheels. Suitcases being dragged like an errant dog, behind a slow moving, travel weary individuals. The only problem it's never an individual. It's never less than three persons. The suitcases are alright when they are being wheeled. But when picked up the true weight of the kitchen sink becomes apparent and it is an almighty struggle to wrestle them onto the train. The very fact that these are commuter trains also becomes clear once the cases are inside. There is absolutely no place for them to be stored.

They sit in the aisle, a clear and present danger for the chins of anyone foolhardy enough to attempt a hurried exit. There are never enough carriages to seat the hordes. It should not appear totally unreasonable or illogical, that the transport services foresee this annual influx and cater for it. It is not as if they don't know it going to happen. It's been happening for years. Yet the arrival of the tourists seems to surprise everyone. This could be the result of the Blair years where the UK could be described, because of foreign policy, as a pariah in the international community.

A Cheerful Depression

Anyway, it was into this mass of seething humanity that I escaped and became anonymous. A palpable feeling of relief, of freedom almost, washed over me. I could breath normally again, albeit a tad toxic. I meandered my way to the railway station to find I had only just missed a train. There would another in 30 minutes and I made my way to the bar. A pint of lager, I hadn't tasted one in weeks. I found a quiet spot, quiet only in that there was no one within two feet of me, and sipped the cold contents of the glass. It was good, it was normal. I managed to block the cacophony of noise surrounding me and re ran the previous hour in my mind while sipping my beer.

Now that I was away from the hotel, the whole thing didn't seem so bad. I thought that, on reflection, I had acquitted myself in an acceptable manner. I couldn't shake the feeling I had that all was not well. I was, I knew, reading the worst into the situation again, forecasting doom and gloom, still envisaging the absolutely worst thing that could possibly happen. I wanted badly to forget this, push it away, but it persisted way after the time I got home and into the evening. By the time I went to bed my return to work had assumed disastrous proportions. This, of course, led to a nearly sleepless night, resulting in the thoughts still being present in the morning. I then had all day for them to grow and worsen. I could not banish them, could not contain or confine them, no matter what I did. Being at the gym only heightened them; it was almost my place of work.

During all this there hadn't been any thoughts of self harm. I appeared to have grown out of that particular phase. I didn't think how breaking my arm would help avoid the inevitable return to work. Although I was in an anxious state I thought I was coping quite well with the prospect. The visit the previous day had served the purpose of breaking back into the environment before submitting myself to a full day. The first day of work should, therefore, be straightforward, easy, to be viewed as a return after some time off.

The anxiety attacks increased the nearer the day approached. I fought them, almost screaming in frustration, I tried to relax, I tried to sleep. Logic told me that I wasn't nearly as bad as I had been, but it didn't feel that way. I was going to start work a wreck, exhausted before I even started. I made myself perform the routine tasks associated with work. Dry cleaning, washing and ironing of shirts, cleaning of shoes. Anything to give me a sense of the mundane.

The night before was sleepless. My mind would not shut down as I anticipated every eventuality the following day could bring. I was relieved to see day light breaking. I could get out of bed and start my morning routine, showering, shaving and dressing before making my way to the station for 06h30.

I would like to be able to tell you that all was well, that I was looking forward to going back, that I was excited and happy at the prospect of seeing friends and colleagues. I wasn't. I was terrified. My mind was playing tricks on me, my body was displaying symptoms of illnesses I couldn't possibly have. But, as with all stories, there has to be a part when all appears to be going reasonably well, when the worst is over, and this is that point in my story. I hoped fervently that this was to be the case, that a return to work would bring me back to normality, that I could forget the last year. In the background, however, huge, towering thunderclouds were gathering. A storm of gigantic proportions was about to be unleashed. I never even saw the darkening horizon.

I never anticipated the horrors that were to invade my mind. I could not know the depths of misery which were lurking around the corner; a dark, malevolent, truly evil, malignant force was lurking in the wings. The curtain was about to go up on an act so terrible it would change my life forever.

CHAPTER 5

The 06h33 train left the station at 06h37, one minute later than the usual lateness. It rolled through the green and pleasant lands that were Central Scotland. The train was, as usual, full. Familiar faces hidden behind newspapers. The same people in the same seats as every morning, talking about the same things. The usual suspects were dozing as they train wound it's way through station after station. The journey was interminable. Outside the door to the hotel I paused for a few minutes to settle myself, gird my loins, gather my thoughts.

Once inside I followed the same routine I had long since adopted. Phase one was going well, the catching up with all the paperwork was soon complete. E-mails read and notes made. Then the walk around the various departments, having a cup of coffee with other managers. Trying to relax, laugh and be interested. I even managed to have a chat to some guests who were sitting in the lounge waiting to go on some excursion or the other. The morning, I thought, was going well. I was getting into the swing of things. I was sure that as the normal routine re-established itself over the coming weeks all would be well.

I wish that something untoward had happened on that first day back at work. But nothing did. It was a quiet day. The business guests had gone to their meetings the tourists had left on the coaches for tours. Everything progressed as it normally had. The deep clean was due to start when I returned from time off. This was a good day to climb back into the saddle. The conferences being held were progressing well. No hiccups. I actually felt superfluous to requirement. I had no special responsibility. I was free to acclimatize myself in whatever way I felt most comfortable with.

Perhaps for this reason the anxiety lessened to a more

controllable, acceptable level. I was still conscious of my thinking that all and sundry were looking at me, knowing my discomfort. This is, of course, absolute nonsense. They all had their own worries and work to do without thinking about me. I was certain that this feeling would pass over the next few days. All in all, as I retired to my office in the afternoon I thought the day had gone as well as could have been expected. Sitting at my desk I experienced the same emotion as before about not being my old self. There did seem to be a part of me that was missing. I didn't know what part of me that was. I had demonstrated that I still had a sense of humor and the ability to make a decision. Just a nagging doubt in my mind that I wasn't the same person. Again I dismissed this. I had to endure a back to work interview with the HR manager. Here I freely admit that I lied through my back teeth about my abilities, refusing to admit to him that I was possibly not ready for a return. It was agreed that I would take it easy, a gradual reintroduction into the areas of responsibility. If, at any time, I felt overwhelmed I was to simply leave and go home. It was all so easy then; there was nothing there that I felt I couldn't handle. I knew I could live with the anxiety attacks; I could take them and stick them where the sun doesn't shine and ignore the feelings of inadequacy. I reasoned that these self doubts may even help me perform my job to higher standards as I strived to fight these doubts.

I wasn't sorry to reach the end of the day. I was pleased, inordinately proud of myself for having attained the goal set. This brought a smile to my face as I thought of how Samuel would react to this. "Quite right," he would say, "you have done well. You did what you set out to do. While there may have been doubts and anxiety you dealt with them. Small goals, steps at a time and in no time you'll be back to where you were."

I resolved to try and remember that, see if he actually did say that at our next appointment.

A Cheerful Depression

A cold beer was my reward to myself as I waited for the train. I tried to block out what I thought others might be saying about me now that I was no longer present and concentrate my mind on the good things that had been achieved. This I have always found to be the hardest task. Sometimes it's hard to plough through the murk and fix your sights on the positives. I worked really hard at this while I finished my beer and then sat on the train. I found I was able to close my eyes and actually felt myself relaxing in the rhythmic movement of the train. This was surely a good sign.

Once inside my apartment I found that I felt exhausted. A result of a full day's work, physical and mental effort catching up on me. A snack and into bed. Bliss, I fell asleep almost immediately. This had been such a rare occurrence that it was to be celebrated in the morning by a slow awakening and an even slower rise from the bed. I felt rested, which, in turn, made me feel more relaxed, more confident. That day surely qualifies as the best day I had experienced for a long, long time. My mood was buoyant, I wanted to go out. As a treat I decided I would take myself for a pub lunch. I had always enjoyed doing something like this on my days off, a break from slaving over a hot stove. But this would be the first time in over a year that I was confident enough to sit for a meal in a public place. I didn't count the meals in the staff canteen as I always went down after the guests had finished their lunch, the result being that most of the time I was on my own anyway. This, while being a deliberate act, had, in my opinion, nothing to do with my condition. It was easier to eat in a relaxed manner knowing that the meal was less likely to be interrupted with a call to sort some problem.

So I went out to my favorite and most frequented pub, a single man's best friends – waiting staff and barmaids. They remembered me despite the long absences and it made for a pleasant distraction for an hour or two, chatting to them, enjoying a burger and chips and a couple of beers. They told me how their studies and various pursuits were progressing. They were really very good kids, they had their ambitions and aspirations, their whole life lay in front of them. Some of them I have known since their high school days, or when they started at university and took a job in the Stirling hotel to earn their keep. Being a small town we were always bumping into each other and they always brought up to date on what had been happening in their lives. Jamie is one who springs to mind, a great young lad with a lot of potential when I first met him during my first job back in the UK when I was the Human Resources Manager for a small hotel and conference center. I tried to guide him, giving him advice to steer him down the right path, to develop his abilities. That, after all was my job. Now, as a man and a success, he insists on introducing me as his mentor, the one who put him on the straight and narrow. This is embarrassing, he did it all himself and, for me, it is extremely gratifying that he took some of my advice and achieved his goals. It is pleasing that, in some small way, you can make a contribution and then see the results first hand. Their enthusiasm and their joie d'vivre is always a pleasure to observe. They made me forget, for a short time, my own misery and self pity.

As I walked home I must admit that I did feel better. The one advantage of these passing and fleeting exchanges was that they were totally unaware of what was happening with my life. For that to have happened I would have to have burdened them with my story and that would not have been fair. I have never subscribed to the theory that a person working behind a bar is a substitute for a psychologist, someone to patiently listen to the woes of the world, how someone's wife doesn't understand them. I feel sorry for any surviving bar staff who still have to conform to this stereotypical view. A good two days. Was normality finally returning? Was I now regaining the ability to cope with the vagaries of my mind?

Alcohol is a depressant, we all know that. Two beers taken

A Cheerful Depression

slowly, over two hours, was not, in my opinion, something that should increase anxiety and it is entirely possible I am wrong in attributing my subsequent low mood to them. Once home I did some work on the computer while listening to the Country and Western radio station. I was not aware of any particular song or other trigger which plunged my mood into the depths. One thing I know now is that it can happen without warning. I tried to keep working, failed and gave up. Then I spent the rest of the evening worrying about the reasons for this sudden and dramatic change in mood. Probably the worst thing I could have done in the circumstances, there was no explanation and the only result was frustration and anger at myself. All the mix of emotions and negative thoughts were back in abundance. The result was yet another poor night's sleep and the continuance of them in the morning. Why? I felt like screaming at the mirror. It was just so bloody frustrating and I didn't know how to rectify it. My sessions with Samuel had not gone that far to this point. I had to hope that it would pass as quickly as it had begun.

Feelings of hopelessness were prevalent throughout that day. I hated vehemently this inability to cope with the smallest task when I was like this. Even going to the bathroom was a mountain to climb on a day like this. I wanted to curl up in bed and pull the duvet over my head. I do not believe that thoughts of work were in any way involved. I do not remember thinking about work in any shape or form. I was too busy concentrating on my misery. I couldn't shake it. I couldn't control it. That is the worst thing, and I have referred to it often, lack of control. During the whole time of the illness I have never felt in control. I have been unable to control my mind, the thought process. I have been unable to control the anxiety and the physical aspect of it. I have been unable to control my sleep and my ability to relax. My lack of control over ineptness to cope with everyday, simple matters was perhaps the most worrying. My coping mechanism was sinking beneath the waves, shot full of more holes than

George Bush's foreign policy.

Things were, for some reason, getting away from me. It felt as if there was too much to deal with. I couldn't rationalize that there was nothing in life which was insurmountable, which could be dealt with by a little application. Under *"normal"* circumstances that would have been the case, a bit of effort and all these petty little problems would have been resolved. Unfortunately that was not how I saw them. They assumed a significance far beyond the actual norm. Each was a mountain that could not be climbed and, together, they formed a mountain range that stretches as far as the eye could see.

Still I fought. I tried to seek solutions. All my efforts were put into pulling my mind together and working things out. It was to no avail. My brain would not focus. It would not provide me with any positive feedback. It produced negative response after negative response. This did not strike me as abnormal. I had become accustomed to this way of thinking over a period of fourteen months. I was not concerned about the negativity of my thoughts. I was concerned about the fact that I could not come up with any solutions to the problems I saw besetting me, weighing me down.

The third day off was slightly better. I felt an acceptance, an inevitability about the whole process. There was no progress with regard to solutions but I had slept nearly the whole night. My mind must have exhausted itself. Now normally, and I suppose it's true for a lot people, I go to sleep with a concern and wake up with the answer. This hadn't happened. I only awoke with the acceptance that there wasn't anything to be done.

I plodded through the chores of the day. I prepared myself for work the day after the next. I was ready to go back, I was planning how I would handle the tasks I had been given. Again there was the acceptance, I would manage. It was as if

A Cheerful Depression

my mind had died or, at best, switched into some form of automatic pilot, performing at its base level.

I had been to do the shopping, food that was required for the next four days when I would be arriving home late and leaving early. My shirts were ironed and hung away. My apartment was clean. I had even splurged and spent a pound on a Lottery ticket for that night.

All these plans had been made. I was going to continue to fight through this thing. I didn't relish the thought of continuing in this manner, but had accepted I had to. After I arrived home I set the video recorder for some programmes later that night. I did not feel that my mood had dropped by any significant level. I was carrying on as I had done before, preparing myself for the days ahead. There didn't, however, seem to be any days ahead which I could look forward to, nothing on which I could pin my hopes or aspirations.

It was late afternoon and I was sitting watching the afternoon movie with my brain as good as dead in my head when the answer was obvious. I switched off the television, went to the fridge and took out a can of lager. I was also lucky enough to have a packet of crisps in the cupboard and took them back to my chair. I put pen to paper and started writing a note, to be read when someone found my body. I intended to kill myself.

On reflection I know that this decision was taken out of despair. Not the kind of despair felt when something goes wrong in life. I have felt the deep sense of loss of a loved one. I have felt the despair of knowing that I would never see them again, the gut wrenching, heart-breaking kind of grief that hurts physically. At the time I vowed that I would never feel like that again. I had, as everyone has, the feeling that the heart is literally breaking, that it would impossible to survive the loss. But this was different. I did not feel any sense of loss, any grief, any pain. It was the despair born of the inescapable fact that nothing could be done, there was no tomorrow. I suppose that was the worst part – I could not see any tomorrow. There would not be a tomorrow and that was a good thing, as far as I was concerned. It is very hard to try and describe these feelings, the fact that there was absolutely and definitely no future, no hope, no escape from the present. I knew there was to be no more joy or happiness in my life. It actually was that simple. There was even a feeling of despair which I had felt before. It was an emptiness, a void, in which I was floating. There was no umbilical cord holding me to reality, to reason.

There was no emotion attached to this decision. I referred to the manner of my death earlier on. Well, I didn't have a bottle of whiskey but I did have two beers, some crisps and cigarettes. The beautiful woman did not matter. I was going to drink the beer and have a last cigarette or two while I wrote a note. I wanted to write a note to try and explain why I was going to do this. Further I didn't want anyone to blame themselves for my taking my life. This was paramount in my mind. I imagined that a few people would regard themselves badly because they didn't see it coming. I tried to explain that they couldn't have seen it coming. I hadn't, at least not until 16h00 that day. The note turned into five pages as I endeavored to cover as much as I could. I know that I said in it that I missed a lot of people and by doing this I would be reunited with them. I believe it was concise and well written. I signed the note and put it on my bedside table. It was 17h25 when I finished this and I resolved to do the deed at 18h00. The old habit of setting a deadline was still prevalent. Funny the way habits take over even in the worst of circumstances.

Sitting, as I finished the second beer and another cigarette I thought what I might do to minimize the mess that would made at the moment of death. The only things I had were towels and I decided to wrap myself in them when I went to bed. I also opened the windows to vent the rooms. As I

A Cheerful Depression

finished I checked the quantity of pills. I knew that a failure might lead to damaged organs but there was the certainty - I would not fail. I had thirty three days of 200mg a day, over 6,000 mg of Seratoline, nineteen sleeping pills and fifteen days worth of something to combat anxiety. I forget what it was called. It was enough to knock down a bull elephant. I was absolutely sure that I would not survive the night. I emptied all my pills into a cup, filled a glass with water, rather irrationally went to the bathroom before undressing and climbing into bed.

Once in bed I wrapped layers of towels around my waist and legs. I had put on a pair of sweats to help with this. I lay back and lit another cigarette, finishing it before taking all the pills, swallowing as much I could at one time, but finishing them all in under a minute. Then I lay back and waited for sleep. I don't remember falling asleep. I remember lying there and looking at the ceiling, aware of the daylight coming through the open curtains, asking myself if I should have closed them, before closing my eyes. My last thought was that at least it was finished. No more pain, no more missing people who I had known and loved, no more recriminations, no more worries. I was content to lie there and die.

I hoped I would not be judged to harshly, nor would there be any pity. This was what I wanted, it was the only way out I could take. That the contents of the note would explain what I was feeling.

The thought of talking to someone prior to this did not cross my mind. There were no second thoughts about the act. From my point of view at the time it was a cold and calculated decision. Why I went to the bother of trying to minimize the mess I don't know. I would be dead. It would be someone else's problem. I assume that is part of the irrational thought process that drives one to commit suicide in the first place. I also know that popular thinking is that taking pills, an overdose, is a woman's way of killing oneself. Well, if I had been in possession of a gun, I would have, in all likelihood, put that in my mouth. I never thought about sitting in the bath and cutting into my wrists. Taking the pills, which I had in abundance, was the logical and reasonable method. Prior to 16h00 there had been no thought of doing this, not consciously at least. Nothing happened that day of any import. I did not cry. I did not ask God's forgiveness. I did not want anything other than to end it all. End what? I don't, to this day, know. Were things so bad? Yes, in my mind things were so bad it was unbearable. Killing myself was the only solution open to me. It would solve everything.

There were no thoughts about how anyone would know what I had done. Who would find me or what would happen when they did find me. I did not think about the next day. Why should I? I would be dead.

There are people who will scoff at this as weakness and mouth words like irrational, desperate. It was those and more. Is it insanity? No it is not insanity. It may feel like. It may sound like it. But no, it is not insanity. It is a shutting down of the ability to cope. It is the knowledge that you have sunk so low into an ocean of despair from which there is no rescue, which drives these thoughts. My decision was a result of fourteen months of battling this insidious disease and losing, for one day, the fight.

My eyes opened. It was daylight. I lay in the same position. I thought I had only closed my eyes for an instant. I turned my head and looked at the clock. It was 07h30. That couldn't be correct. It was. I moved on the bed and felt a wetness covering me from my waist to my knees.

Then I knew. I was not dead. It was a terrible, horrific feeling. I couldn't believe I was still alive. I didn't want to be alive. It is the most devastating, overwhelming feeling of disappointment that I have ever experienced. I lay still and closed my eyes, hoping beyond hope that death would still come, that this was merely an aberration in the process. I tried to convince myself that I could still die. I had after all voided both my bladder and bowels. I could feel the contents against my skin. Still nothing happened. I could not go back to sleep. I cried. This was not how it was meant to be. Now I had to face another day, the same fears, nothing had changed. Even with all those pills inside me I still felt the same despair.

I had to get up. I knew I couldn't lie there in my filth. Those old habits again. It took a long time for me to clean myself and then start on the bed. Fortunately the protective layers had done the job. Everything was confined to the towels and easily placed in bin liners to be disposed off. I stripped the bed and put everything in the wash. Now I was clean again I knew I had to phone someone. I did not feel particularly well, I was unsteady, my legs felt like rubber.

Of course, this was only to be expected. I had punished my body with the amount of pills. It was 09h00 by the time I had finished the cleansing process and I called my GP first. After I had explained to him what I had done he told me to wait as he was sending an ambulance. I then phoned Samuel to tell him. I don't know why I did this. Possibly he had become someone I could trust, someone who would not condemn me outright for my action. Aside from the fact that I was beginning to feel terribly unwell, I do not have an explanation for these phone calls. I wanted to die yet I phoned for assistance. Possibly the fact that I survived my attempt and was, somehow, realizing, perhaps subconsciously, that I needed help made me do it. I do know that I wasn't thinking straight, I was performing on instinct. I managed to pack an overnight bag and waited on the ambulance. They were very quick in their response; I had barely hung up after speaking to Samuel. They wanted to put me in a chair to get me out to their vehicle but I insisted on walking, weakly and unsteady but walk unaided I did. The effort almost did for me; I needed their help to climb into the ambulance. Stubborn, old fool.

They noted what I had taken. I am not sure if I was as coherent as I thought I was being, but we managed to get all the details down before arriving at the hospital.

Now I had to deal with the consequences of my actions. I had no idea what to expect when I got to the hospital. Part of me didn't even want to be there. Once there I did require help. I had difficulty in standing. They wheeled me in, sat in a wheelchair, past what felt like crowds of people, all staring at me. I looked at my hands, they were yellow, my skin was yellow, but it was a distracted thought. I was looking down at myself, from the outside. I was placed on a bed in the emergency room and I started to lose it. I was becoming disorientated and wanting to sleep. I was aware of the doctor talking to me asking me questions which I tried to answer. I was attached to monitors; I remember her telling me that the amount I had taken could adversely affect the heart. Good news seeped through the mesh shielding my brain. Maybe I could still die. But I wasn't, by now, in any condition to notice much. I must have given the doctor Mary's phone number as she turned up, standing at the side of the bed holding my hand. I recall her asking who had been called but I didn't know and she said she would go and call work and my sister. I drifted in and out of this daze the whole morning. No awareness of the passage of time or what was happening around me, always the hope that my heart would stop. I wanted to tell them not to revive me if that happened, but I kept forgetting. Why, oh, why do they not have euthanasia for people like me? I would gladly have been treated like a horse with a broken leg – they shoot horses don't they? I was definitely not in the best position to decide my treatment. The only certainty was, still, the desire for it all to end, that and the bitter disappointment that I was laying in hospital. It really was a terrible day.

A Cheerful Depression

Every time I came round Mary was there, I know I talked to her, she told me she had phoned work and my sister. She left saying she would return in the evening. It is all very vague. But, as the day wore on, X rays were taken, the thought that I was there was wasting everyone's time began to bother me. I didn't deserve the treatment, the care. I had tried to kill myself. God I couldn't even manage that successfully. I was now officially a waste of time and energy. It was confirmation. I hated myself with a vengeance. How could these doctors and nursing staff take time to talk to me, look after me and be nice to me? I wanted to escape but I couldn't. I had tried to sit up on my own for the X ray and failed miserably. How was I going to escape? I wasn't. This would be the first part of my punishment, the consequence of failure. Oh, how badly I hoped that something, anything would go wrong. This whole episode was inconceivable. I could not reconcile the fact that I did not die. I must have been close at some stage. Why not that final slip? What had pulled me back? It most certainly was not the desire to go on living.

At least in the ward I was given a private room. I couldn't have faced anyone. The inevitable questions. It was better for me to wallow alone in my misery. And that's all I did. I lay, unmoving staring at the ceiling and thinking. Why was I still alive? That was the predominant thought, pushing all else aside in it's persistence.

I wouldn't describe as what I did over the next fifteen hours as sleep. It was a drifting in and out of awareness. I would have dearly liked to escape for a short while into sleep but it wasn't to be. Mary did return at some point in the evening. Maybe it was me but she seemed scared. Scared of me, of what I had done. It was an uncomfortable visit and I am sure that this was all in my tortured imagination. It took a long time before daylight started lighting the window and the bustle of shift changeover at the nursing station began. I managed to get up and shower. A welcome relief. It felt good to be clean. The memory of the mess from the preceding morning still clear in my mind and I scrubbed and scrubbed until I was sure every last vestige was gone. The scrubbing may have had some psychological aspect, but I am not qualified to comment on that.

I had a visit from a psychiatric nurse who assessed me and then said she was calling a group called IHTT, intensive home therapy, who would come and see prior to my discharge. I managed to convince everyone that I was fine and capable of looking after myself when I got home. I was sure there would no repeat of the suicide attempt. I think I was so high on the drugs remaining in my system that I would have said anything to get out of there.

My last visitor prior to my release was the priest I had asked for the previous night. We had a chat and I told him what I had done and the reasons why. I asked that he hear my confession which he did, giving me the absolution I needed. It was a major issue for me – surviving a suicide attempt – to try this and to succeed is a cardinal sin. By confessing, at least one aspect of my guilt was alleviated in some small measure. I only had the other 99.99% to deal with. I honestly had no idea, not even the vaguest concept, as to how I was going to move forward after this. I was utterly defeated. I could not find an ounce of strength to fight anymore.

Once home I sat and tried to think. I found I couldn't think of anything apart from the fact that I was a failure of greatest magnitude. I couldn't bear to look at myself in the mirror. I loathed what I had become. No matter what, I could not move myself from my chair. In the evening my mind wandered into the realms of the insurmountable problems which I still faced. They appeared to me to be even more impossible to resolve than they had before. I did contemplate running a bath and trying the whole process again, this time by cutting my wrists. What stopped me? The thought of failing again prevented me

A Cheerful Depression

from doing anything.

That was the only reason, another failure in, what I saw, a long line of failings. This torment was to continue for weeks. I couldn't resolve any of the issues facing me. I couldn't kill myself. The downward spiral had ceased. It could drop no more. I was at rock bottom with no way out. In a pit with walls so smooth there was not even a toe hold. I was trapped in a prison of my own making.

I found the lottery ticket I had purchased. On checking the numbers I saw that I had won £10. What a supreme irony it would have been had I won the jackpot but had succeeded in my attempt on my life!

Then, joy of joys. I had acquired an infection while I had been in hospital. My left forearm from the elbow down was infected, discolored and swollen. During the daily visit I was advised, no I was instructed, to go to the GP. I did so and was prescribed antibiotics. I did take the whole course.

What I didn't tell anyone was that I tried to worsen the infection. I would tie a belt tightly around my upper arm, a tourniquet, to restrict the flow of blood to the lower arm and hand. I would hold on until my hand turned blue, then a darker hue. What I hoped to achieve is beyond me. If I had succeeded in doing anything it may have resulted in the loss of my arm. I never told anyone I did this and, should Samuel and the others read this, I will undoubtedly be in trouble. I continued this practice for a week with no result and then stopped it as quickly as I had begun. I think that I wanted something physiologically wrong with me, not an unseen, mental problem, rather something I could see and feel. After this I felt pathetic, stupid and ashamed.

I was visited daily through this period by a psychiatric nurse from the IHTT. He brought my medication and stayed and talked with me. I am ashamed to admit that I cried frequently in front of him. He never judged me. He tried to guide me, gently pushing me in the correct direction where I could start to feel that I regaining some control of my life. Without knowing that I was doing the right thing I started to, again, take myself outside whenever dark thoughts started to prevail.

A week after the attempt I was standing making a cup of coffee in the kitchen. This was one of those moments when realization strikes. I had been, as usual, been feeling worthless and thinking how much of a fraud I was, all the effort people were taking over me. Out of the blue, and I said it out loud, I knew that I was ill. I had, after all tried to kill myself. I couldn't cope with life. I couldn't deal with the smallest things in my life. *I was ill.* This in itself was a significant moment as I had never admitted to myself or anybody that I was ill. I had refused to accept it. The fact that I couldn't see, hear or touch this illness had always been an inhibiting factor for me.

Did this make an immediate difference to my thinking? No, not in the least. It did make me more receptive to measures which would help my recovery. That was the most important aspect it, acceptance of the professional help that was available.

Slowly, oh so very slowly, I became less dependent on the daily visits. I had seen Samuel and we had talked the episode through. I had asked about a Benefits and Debt adviser who worked with the Mental Health unit. An appointment was set to have a look at my financial situation which was by now in disarray. I had completely ignored it, letters remained unopened. The phone had remained unanswered. The time had passed with nothing being done. Now the finances were a cause of concern on top of everything else. I must point out that in normal times it would not have been a major factor, phone calls would have resolved all and a small amount of effort could have taken care of things. As it happened this is

A Cheerful Depression

what Charlie did. He took the burden from my shoulders and helped obtain forms for claiming payment protection insurance. He did not remove all responsibility from me, how could he, I still had to work out what was what.

It was a step in the right direction. Remembering our first meeting I was like a cat on a hot tin roof. I couldn't settle down, I couldn't retain thoughts in any logical sequence. He wouldn't let me abdicate all my responsibility.

Unfortunately, I was now receiving Statutory Sick Pay from my employer which was no where nearly enough to cover the basics. I had forgotten, more likely ignored, that aspect. When I went to the bank to draw money on pay day, the amount paid in was minuscule in comparison to my normal salary. I went straight back to go, I didn't collect the £200, there wasn't that much in my account. I dropped right back to the bottom, hell, I had barely made an upward move, so the drop didn't hurt that much. It was to have been the last home visit, however, when he saw me he put that on hold. I was a wreck. Again, I was in the position where I didn't know which to turn. I could not cope. I could not think. He managed to settle me down to a more rational level.

I had to ask for help from somewhere. I had to phone my sister and see if she could lend me some money to cover the basics. Rent, electricity and such. He helped me do this. It was horrible, after a brief chat to her. He took the phone back as I had broken down completely. However, it did ease the strain a bit, gave me some breathing space.

I did speak with Mona again briefly but could not bring myself to discuss the illness over the phone. I wrote a long e-mail detailing all that had happened. I covered it all, in a way it was a relief, conversely it was also a cause for concern. I worried that she in turn would worry and, because of the worry, pester me. That is not a nice word to use when someone who cares tries to help and maintain contact, but that was how I looked at the intrusion into my world. I had also completely bared my soul to someone other than a health worker and it left me feeling vulnerable.

There was something I, and only I could do. I had to speak to my boss and resign from work. The financial constraints were the primary reason for this, but there was also the concern that my recovery would take a while and I didn't want my colleagues placed under pressure covering for me for a long period. I arranged to meet him and put this to him. It was the first time I had seen anyone since the attempt and I had dig up my public face. I put a lot of effort into appearing normal. I did not cry or break down in front of him, as a result of a testing exercise in self control. I wrote a letter of resignation. That was that. Another aspect of pressure had been removed. I didn't have to concern myself about a date to return to work. The worry about how others at work would be viewing my ongoing illness was removed.

Extract from my journal at the time:

Woke up feeling a bit more relaxed than have done lately. Trying to stay relaxed about the day ahead and stop catastrophising about the visit to the hotel and the train ride. Looking at the day ahead everything seems so difficult and tasks insurmountable, even folding the laundry. Sense of dread about everything - feel threatened but do not know what I'm scared of. Even keep forgetting what I want to put down in here - for example I am still all fumbling and shaky even at home. I forget what I'm doing as my mind wanders off on a tangent, this is all day and is especially frustrating when I'm trying to sleep. Went through to hotel, anticlimax after all anxiety. Felt ok after leaving but took bad again at home, felt as if no-one cares I have left or how I am. Really making myself feel down, cannot wait to go to bed and escape.

A Cheerful Depression

It was progress of sorts. The principal concern in these weeks was to remove as much pressure as I could from myself. To give myself some breathing space to concentrate on getting well. But still my inability to cope was a strong issue keeping me down. I still hated myself. I still viewed myself as a failure. The steps I had taken only confirmed this. I needed help to sort out my finances,

I had to leave my job. I could not cope with the day to day requirements of living. Worse of all, my fate, my future was now in the hands of others. The health professionals, the DWP for benefits, there was very little I could do to control my own life, to control my thoughts.

Six weeks after the suicide attempt I was to see Charles, the psychiatrist, again. This time he altered my medication completely. Now I was to take Mirtazapine at night, this would help me sleep he said. The night terrors had increased in frequency again and were horrendously vivid and disturbing. The ability to have a good sleep would improve my outlook. After I had completed the changeover and reached the required dosage he would start another pill to help me through the day.

Woke up and thought "Oh no, not another day, I bloody survived the night again." Not that I had done anything to not survive. It was an f...cking awful night again, waking up almost every hour until 3 then slept until about 6 and got up at 07h30. Immediately felt low when I woke up, no point to anything. What shit is this day going to bring? - Extract from journal.

I really wanted, needed, the night terrors to stop. I was struggling to differentiate between dreams and reality. Everyday objects in the bedroom assumed nightmare dimensions, incorporated as they were into the dream or the period of waking. The dreams were generally full of extreme violence, in places only an imagination can produce. Sometimes the surroundings, the faces were familiar but they were out of context with what had actually happened. Now I can think back to these dreams and wish I had written down the contents. They would have made a good horror movie.

I also hoped that the new medication would help with my concentration which had again slipped to a new low. My mind would go off on a tangent. I could sit for hours, my mind being blown in different directions, swirling, twisting and turning, playing tricks on my consciousness. These *"daydreams"* could be as distracting and as confusing as the night terrors. Again it was sometimes hard to distinguish between reality and the daydream. Not too pleasant if you think you've won the lottery only to find it was a daydream. Fortunately, I never experienced that extreme, but there were similar scenarios. I tried to read during this time but found it frustrating as I would have to turn back pages to find the last part I could remember. A book I could normally have finished in two or three days, now took weeks.

I was still seeing my key worker, Samuel, during this time. He remained positive and optimistic, always able to find something in my existence which was good. The fact I had given up work was good, I had taken control over that aspect of concern. The fact I was trying to sort out finances was also a positive sign, again I was doing something for myself. I, of course, did not see these things in the same light, it still reeked of failure. On my way to see him I would rack my brains to think of something about which I tell him. In retrospect I suppose this was the whole object of the exercise. I was being forced to think on my own, deliberately concentrating on the good happening to me, no matter how small. I took to making notes on my mood, my feelings and how I felt on a daily basis. This was designed principally to try and remember things. I was having terrible problems with my memory and the lack of concentration which I have already mentioned. There were times when I dreaded going to see Samuel. Mainly due to the fact that I had struggled to come up with a positive.

Although, sometimes it was plain and simple, I didn't want to go out, even if it was for my own benefit. However, I did manage to make all the appointments. I was inordinately proud of this. If, for some reason, I was unable to go, I would phone and change the date. Again, this very tiny step can be viewed as progress of sorts.

I had completely withdrawn from everyone. I resented someone phoning. I did not want to go out, even for a walk. I did not see any point in doing any of these things. Was I trying to protect myself? I do know I was continuously worried about the delicate state of my mind. Samuel and Ian have told me that there is a strong survival instinct inside me, which possibly explains why I didn't die from the overdose. I am sure that we all have this primeval instinct, the fight or flight feelings we all experience are part of it. It is a natural part of the brain telling us what to do to survive in any given situation. Perhaps it was this that made me concerned about my fragile state, an unconscious unwillingness to let go again, to revert back to the stage where killing myself was the one and only option left open to me. It may very well be this introspective aspect of my thinking that prevented any further self harm.

Once the letter from my employer arrived with the effective final date of employment the next hurdle was to register a claim for benefit. I had the whole weekend to think about it. I reduced myself to constant state of anxiety and worry over this. I planned the whole thing in my head. I foresaw every aspect; I *knew* that it was all going to go badly for me. You would think that with this new found ability to forecast the future I could have started a new job as a psychic. It's just as well I didn't, my every prediction of disaster was wrong. I mentioned this to Samuel and he gave a new word for this – *catastrophising.* Forecasting, knowing the worst that was bound to happen in any given situation. I suppose we all do this to a certain extent. It can be useful, thinking the worst and then being pleasantly surprised when things don't turn out as badly as we had thought. It's much the same with anxiety.

Everyone becomes anxious over everyday events, a job interview, for example. The difference with a depressive illness is that these normal thoughts become blown out of all proportion. They assume such a negative, distorted aspect as to become destructive. They take over and rapidly become the norm. A cycle that is harder to break than the smoking habit. This negativity destroys self esteem and self-confidence. They produce doubts with regard to one's ability to deal with simple problems, and subsequently the doubt becomes a reality, a fact. Hiding from them is easier than failing to deal with them.

Goal setting was an important part of my everyday life. One goal was to get up. Another would be to go out, to the shop or for a walk. To deal with the Job Center. Not to achieve any of these goals was to fail and attribute an inordinate amount of blame on one's self. To compliment yourself on achieving even the smallest of goals was important. It may sound silly to tell yourself you have done well in making it to the shop, even though beset with anxiety and fear, but it is important. You have succeeded. You did what you set out to do. An achievement. All this is very easy to say. It is infinitely harder to do. At the time, complimenting yourself on being able to go to the shop, is ludicrous, asinine in the extreme.

What of the recovery process? These small steps in the weeks following the suicide attempt were the start of the recovery. The tunnel I was in was a dark and foreboding place with no light, not even a glimmer, at the other end. But I had taken the first steps. There has to be a beginning and, although it was

A Cheerful Depression

hard to realize at the time, this was it. I had started. In the same way as an alcoholic cannot be helped until they admit they have a drinking problem, I could not help myself until I admitted that I was ill, albeit a mental illness. A biochemical imbalance in the brain.

I knew, even at this early stage, that I would never be the same person as I had been. I didn't know how I would change, but I knew that change I would.

Possibly it was time to move things on a bit, step up a gear. Samuel had told me about the various groups they held and I now resolved to try and overcome my apprehension and attend one. I resolved to discuss this with him at our next meeting.

Another extract from journal:

This discussing private feelings and emotions in public is not for me. Perhaps, however, it will work and something will be learned from it. A bit weepy again today, tied in with high anxiety levels??? Felt guilty again about my current position and had to remind myself that I did make an attempt to kill myself and that my emotional state is fragile, my coping mechanism does not seem to be working at full power yet either, too many little things upset me too quickly.

CHAPTER 6

Extract from my journal:

God what a bad night, fell asleep around 22h45, woke 00h10, slept and woke at 03h15. Felt sick with an upset stomach. Went to toilet and then was up rest of the night, not tired but getting really fed up with this. Why am I worrying about going to see Samuel? I'm already getting worked up about that. It's not good feeling so down so early in the day. This is a really bad anxiety attack, the more time goes on I actually feel physically ill, as if I want to vomit. In an effort to get over this I have done some cleaning and am actually ready to go at 07h30. This is the WORST it's been for a long time. Don't think I've actually wanted to throw up before. Cannot be anything I had to eat, it wasn't much but it was fresh. It's now 08h00 and I am sooooo tired, I wish I could go back to bed - reaction to having to go out to see Samuel? It's funny because I feel so miserable, physically and mentally - now I'm feeling all weepy, and it's just the morning news!! God knows what will happen if I listen to the radio or watch a movie. God I'm such a loser and wimp.

My visits to the hospital and talks with Samuel continued. I kept going with the effort of trying to see positives about the days in between the visits. However, as you can see from the above there were times when all was not well. The weepy feeling was, I believe, down to a low mood, which in turn was related to the lack of sleep and tiredness. The physical aspects of it can now be explained by the tenseness of the muscles caused by the increasing levels of anxiety. I suggested to Samuel that I thought I might be ready to join a group which would be dealing with Managing Anxiety. I've said before that I did not particularly want to sit in groups of strangers and discuss these feelings, but I agreed. I was willing to try anything. I had been isolated for so long that the just the

A Cheerful Depression

thought of meeting others was terrifying, I did not entertain the thought that I would involve myself in any discussions or whatever they got up to in these sessions. The fear of the unknown crept into my thinking and I was again catastrophising everything, trying to imagine what it would be like.

I really believed that the opinion I had of myself would be mirrored in the opinion others had of me. I was not sure that I was ready to face that. One thing was certain – I had absolutely nothing to lose and everything to gain. My attendance would be viewed by Samuel as a plus – confronting fear head on.

I have never been an advocate of groups of people congregating to discuss abstract issues. I am in favour of such groups, meetings, when they have specifics to discuss and a tangible result at the end. These types of meeting are more than necessary in an age where individuals do not communicate effectively with each other. E mail having taken that away from us. The rest are, in my humble opinion, however, a waste of time. Each person required to attend these is admonished well in advance to prepare themselves by reading the material to be discussed. If these individuals were in possession of half a brain and the ability to read, why then the necessity to sit and be told about it. The meeting will be the most senior person going through all the facts which have become familiar to all. In my opinion this is grandstanding. A need to reinforce the company policy, to drive home his or her importance, a belief held only by the individual and a few others. No argument or dissent is permitted. How can anyone dare to question the word of God? There then follows a spell where self centered little pricks curry favor by re-stating all that had been mentioned previously, sometimes changing the words, more than often, not. Demonstrating how avidly they follow the company line and hang on every word the senior person utters. This is generally accompanied by no small amount of self praise when they describe how they performed to the good of the company and the boss in particular. Those who sit quietly are drawn into making comments that are superfluous to requirement. Anyone who vocalizes a new concept or an opinion which does not conform is then subject to ritual humiliation.

If anyone ever bothered to look back in the minutes, provided, of course, that they were accurately kept, it could be seen that these same opinions and concepts, subtly, or not so subtly altered, often resurface as the original idea of one of the ass kissing yes men/women, several meetings later. It is sometimes amusing to point this out. The reaction is always one of shock. The subject is changed rapidly and the mention is never recorded in the minutes. Fortunately for these self important individuals the person who made the suggestion in the first place has generally left the company, finding it has no place for innovation and his talents. It makes one wonder if the fact that the realization that ambitions and capabilities were incompatible would it be acknowledged or would it ever come to a point where they collide, with the capabilities coming off a poor second. These individuals are easily recognized. They have their name written on the soles of their shoes. This facilitates easy recognition when they are too far up the bosses' backside to see their features.

Anxiety Management – how can you manage anxiety? It happens, it controls you, it takes on a physical form. While extremely nervous I will admit to being intrigued. It never crossed my mind that the others would be in the position as I found myself. I had been dealing with it on my own for so long, I believed I was the only person suffering.

Due to the fact that I respect the privacy and feelings of the others in the group I will not mention any names or any specific comments or reactions. Suffice to say that we all felt the same emotions. We all suffered from almost identical

A Cheerful Depression

fears and insecurities. They were, if you like a mirror into my own soul, a reflection of my own torment. I began to appreciate that I was not alone; my feelings were not unique, belonging to me alone. This alone was a disturbing but, at the same, comforting aspect of the group.

I have to; at this point go into some background for the simple reason that, if you have never experienced these levels of anxiety, it requires some explanation. Now, as we all know, anxiety is an everyday part of life. It can help performance, for example in giving a presentation; it makes us alert before the symptoms recede. Anxiety becomes a problem when it begins to overwhelm, feeling anxious for no reason and is blown out of proportion. This anxiety can cause the body and mind to over-react to everyday situation, making them feel threatening, situations such as waiting in queues, traveling on a bus, being with friends or leaving the house. These events are not a normal reaction. The interaction between the body, brain and behavior create a vicious circle. They all feed into each other, releasing more adrenalin and making you feel worse and feeding upon itself, keeping the whole cycle going. For example; the body can react by sweating and headaches, this in turn feeds the behavior, avoiding doing things, going out, is a good example, and then the brain, it produces thoughts such as, I'll never manage, everyone will stare at me.

As I've said before my symptoms were manifested in the form of chest pain and shortness of breath. However, these can change from person to person and can include nausea, sweating, almost anything you can think of. The most important thing that I had learned was that I was not imagining these feelings, they weren't phantoms, they were real and caused by the amount of adrenalin being released into my body.

In the group we soon found out that we were all experiencing physical symptoms. All these were as real to us as a broken bone, and just as painful. All had experienced poor sleep patterns and feelings of low self worth. People stared at us in shops, avoided us, which increased our anxiety levels. Most of us also felt that, some of the time we were outside ourselves looking in. I have mentioned being awake yet involved in a *daydream, b*eing unable to distinguish dream from reality.

This is a common thing with anxiety – depersonalization – and can last for hours. I personally did not feel fuzzy headed or spaced out when it happened, I felt remote, running on automatic. The one thing we all had in common was avoidance. Avoidance of public places, meeting people; we experienced high levels of anxiety before and during these events. If forced into a one of these then a quick escape was required. The flight or fight response kicking in. All this can develop into phobias, a fear of crowded places, avoidance of one-to-one conversations. I have a phobia in that I have a totally irrational fear of snakes> I can recount many instances when my reactions to the proximity of snakes has been, to say the least, extreme.

When I talked earlier about going to supermarket early in the morning it was to avoid the necessity of queues and the proximity of others. I started the physical symptoms of anxiety a long time before I went out and believed that others were watching me at the check out. I started fumbling, I couldn't open the carrier bags, I felt as if my hand had five thumbs. The longer I was there the worse I felt the worse fumbling became. There were times when I did think I would have to drop everything and leave the shop. Because of this I did not want to go back. I, of course, had to, there was no other alternative. I suppose this can be best described as "fear of fear". I knew what my reaction was going to be and I became scared of it, before it even happened.

We were all in the same boat. It was good to find this out and

A Cheerful Depression

discuss our own ways of dealing with it. Because of the nature of the course and the content there were occasions when the tears flowed. It was really hard to deal with the subjects, but we all persevered. We were all susceptible to these needs to cry, it is hard to discuss how we see ourselves, purely because we do not see ourselves in the same light as they do. We performed an exercise where each of us wrote down a comment about the person next to us and passed it around. When it came back, I know I was surprised, same as everyone about the positive comments made about myself. We simply didn't see those attributes when we thought about ourselves. It is amazing, that we can see the good points in those around us, and are willing to tell them about it, but cannot accept that we are as good.

I gained a great respect for the others in the group who were combating the same illness. After all I knew exactly how they felt! The main difference was that the others had children, families, to look after even when they were feeling at their worst. They had to perform the daily routine of taking children to school, cooking and cleaning and, in some cases, work. How they coped with all that and the illness is beyond me. These women displayed a courage that staggers belief. Courage which is of the highest order in that knowing your fears and insecurities and getting out of bed on a daily basis, despite the fact that your mind is screaming at you to hide, and confronting these fears head on deserves nothing but praise.

I should not have been surprised to find that the majority of the group was women. There was another guy at the start but he, for whatever reason, dropped out. Why should it not have come as a surprise? Well, we guys are not very good at getting in touch with our emotions and even worse at expressing them. We find it hard to concede to a weakness, we have to conform to the concepts that are imposed on us by society. However, it doesn't really matter what you are, bread winner, macho super sportsman, high powered executive; depression can strike anyone at anytime. As difficult as it is to express these fears and feelings even to the GP, it has to be done. I know that everyone sees erratic sleep patterns, loss, or gain in appetite, irritability and self doubts as a integral part of modern life and the pressures we subject ourselves to, but if they start to take on proportions greater than normal then there is potentially a problem developing.

You are probably familiar with the question – if a tree falls in a forest and there is no one around to hear it, does it mean it makes no sound? Apply that principle to the question – if someone is feeling mental anguish and no one sees it, does it mean that the anguish doesn't exist? Men, in particular are very good at hiding things. We think that it will pass with time; we have to go on, deal with it. However, it serves no useful purpose, if anything it is, no matter how hard we try, destructive. No matter how hard we try it must affect our every day lives. The irritability can cause problems at work and home. The poor sleep affects the ability to perform at the optimum level, it's only natural. As I've said – a vicious downward spiral.

Now I had already accepted that I was ill. By attending this group I was recognizing the need to change problem behaviors. The purpose of this group was to help us decide to change and to take steps to challenge the current cycle of behavior, then, most importantly to help us to maintain the changes.

This is where the goal setting comes in. We set ourselves small, achievable goals. The fact that we turned up for the group at all was an achievement. I found, along with everyone else, that the anxiety levels on the morning of the group were high. This despite the fact that the venue was a safe and secure place. *Achievable* is the key word here. It was important to achieve the goals that had been set, for me

A Cheerful Depression

anyway, not achieving them was tantamount to failure. If I failed then I suffered at my own hand, beating myself up, fueling the anxiety and the downward spiral.

It was amazing how quickly we got to know each other. I would imagine that sitting for hours baring your soul, your previously hidden fears and concerns goes a long way on this road. We had all experienced the feeling that we were making an improvement and had slipped back to the beginning bringing on further anxiousness. I know I recounted one of my experiences when I had been writing a novel all morning and had felt that I had completed a particularly good section. I felt really great about myself and what I had done. I left the computer to make a cup of coffee and phone Mary to tell her. However, after talking to her and finishing the coffee, I went on a nose dive into a really low mood. It was all worthless, I had wasted my time, the effort was meaningless. I am not aware of any reason for this slip. It was frustrating and affected me for days, feeding on itself, not allowing me time to pick myself up.

I was lucky in that Samuel was the facilitator of the group and I was able discuss all the points raised and my reactions to them. It was also handy to get his feedback on my handling of the group situation and the degree of involvement. He, as always, remained positive, always reminding me of the good things, explaining away the bad.

There were times when, as I walked home, or sitting at home, I felt that my contribution had been worthless. That the comments and observations I had made were at best asinine, worst puerile.

Diet came through strongly as an important aspect of controlling anxiety and depression. Long periods without eating can reduce the blood sugar levels. Therefore, eating regularly, small amounts every four hours can help. Relaxing while eating, sitting quietly is the best way. To grab a snack and continue working is not as healthy. It cannot only affect your stress levels, but, as in a recent survey, it can damage your health further by contributing to the diseases that accumulate on the keyboard! Definitely better to get away from the desk and eat.

I have looked into diet in an effort to help myself in recovery. Did you know, the naturally occurring substance in chocolate called *phenylethylamine* has been found to elevate endorphin levels and to act as a natural antidepressant? For me this is marvelous news – I love chocolate. It is what I treat myself to when I think I've done something well.

Some vitamins B6, B12 and folate may all help certain forms of depression. B6 in particular has a role in converting trytophan to serotonin in the brain. Trytophan is found in poultry, milk, nuts (including peanuts), eggs and pumpkin seeds. There are of course, many more foods that contain trytophan. This amino-acid is needed to make the mood critical neurotransmitter serotonin. As with everything there can be a down side to the appetite - weight loss or gain. A class of antidepressant drugs called selective serotonin re uptake inhibitors can reduce the appetite, leading to a slight but progressive weight loss. It may be necessary to consult your doctor to find out if this is the case. A special effort may be required to maintain your optimum weight. On the other hand tricyclic antidepressants my cause weight gains.

I have found that there are "feel good" meals which calm and relax me. These meals include carbohydrates in the form of pasta, breads, grains, cereals, fruit and juices. I do not want to go on forever about diet, I am not a dietitian, but I think it is a fact that it can help, if only to make you feel better for the time you are eating. It's keeping that regular, small amounts going that is important. I do know that, when *The Beast* is awakened and is prowling around my brain, that I become

A Cheerful Depression

lethargic and unwilling to make something to eat. The fact that I do, can be regarded as an achievement, something to be celebrated, and it does make me feel better. Besides, if you work it out, cooking a meal is now cheaper than buying a liter of petrol. That's Samuel's influence in seeing the good, coming to the fore! As a point of interest Winston Churchill used to call his bouts of depression as a visit by the *"Black Dog"*.

Possibly the most important of all is the ability to think positively and challenge all those unhelpful thoughts that continually crop up. This is far easier to say that to do. It is possibly the hardest challenge I have had to cope with. The bad feelings became entrenched in my brain. When I found that I could not cope with a task, when I failed in reaching a goal, I became very negative about myself. My anxiety levels increased to a painful degree. All the points that were made during the group were impossible to complete. Even trying a simple thing like taking deep, controlled breathes was an insurmountable task. Knowing that the others were suffering in the same way was of little or no comfort. It was uncomfortable and I felt that I would never rid myself of these feelings.

I had even been subject to the anxiety during the group sessions. A subject which I wanted to shy away from would bring it on. Although I discussed this with Samuel afterwards and he had been aware of my discomfort, it would haunt me for days after, sometimes lasting until the next session, making attendance even harder. At times I wanted to give up, crawl into a corner and hide. Perfectly normal, I was assured, I would work my way through it.

So there we were. We now understood the reasons for the levels of anxiety which we were experiencing. We knew that certain foods could assist in the recovery. We were told about, and practiced breathing exercises and ways to banish the negative thoughts by challenging them and using more positive, more pleasant thoughts to counteract them. I try this method, particularly at night, when I am trying to sleep. I remove myself to a place and concentrate on it, picture the scenery, the smells and the feeling of warmth. Other thoughts try to push their way in and it is hard to stop them. I know that if I permit it, they will become jumbled and confused. They will start racing into a plethora of disturbing images, which will end up with a return of the night terrors.

During the day I found that the secret to keeping negativity at bay was to try and keep my mind busy. This also served the purpose of tiring me. I started writing. I wrote a novel in which I tried to put down on paper my feelings. It was a fictional story, however, the expressions of emotions were real, something I had kept hidden. It was a way of releasing them for the first time, confronting them. Attributing these feelings to an imaginary character was relatively easy. I wasn't describing myself, after all. It was, at times very hard to express myself in this manner, but I persevered and did complete the book. I haven't done anything with it, I suppose I am still afraid of the feeling that rejection will produce. I do not have the self belief to allow anyone else to read it, preferring to believe myself that it is good, without risking the criticism to spoil the dream. If that book is ever published, it will undoubtedly boost my self esteem to levels somewhere near where I used to be.

Anyway, the fact was that this kept me busy for eight, sometimes more, hours a day. My mind was occupied with a task and I was dealing with my emotions, to a degree. It is strange, the feeling I had when I wrote the last line of that first book. I felt empty. I had lost something in my daily routine. I think that quite possibly a part of me went into that book, figuratively speaking, of course. Was it cathartic? I think it was. I believe the expressions of emotion, of love, grief and fear, now being out in the open was beneficial. They had been expressed more vividly in the writing than would ever have been possible in a vocal manner. I would like to think that, when I have made a full recovery, I will be in a better position to express my emotions, without fear of ridicule or of being hurt in the process.

As the group completed the six weeks, we all felt we had been given some tools, some skills with which we could start to manage our anxieties. It had been stated at the start that it was not an overnight fix. That would have been wonderful, but totally unrealistic. I have used the skills on a daily basis. Sometimes I don't even know I'm doing it. But that was the whole point, I understand now, to reach a point where negative feelings can be challenged almost automatically. There are often times when this is not the case and a conscious effort is required and even that don't help. Even in the lowest of times, however, there is the knowledge that although there has been a setback, it is never as bad as it had been. If you keep reminding yourself of this solid fact it does make the low times that little bit easier to deal with.

The struggle continued, even having a better understanding of the enemy and the strategies to confront it, did not make life any easier. In the beginning the knowledge, if anything, made it harder to deal with. There was the knowledge, the expectation, that it could be dealt with, but at the same time there was the certainty that it was a formidable foe that could not be defeated. That was the start of the real battle with anxiety.

Woke up more refreshed, bit of anxiety first thing. Anxious all day, really got uncomfortable, physically and mentally. Kept thinking that I couldn't go on like this, and that there was absolutely nothing left in life for me - no future at all. Felt very down all day and by evening was totally down and felt terrible physically. Had trouble going to sleep but did and slept for two hours. Very fumbly and shaky all day. Extract from journal.

Hours and days were spent locked in combat with my own mind. The results were not encouraging. I would lose time after time. I would become discouraged and disheartened. I was tough on myself on what I regarded as failure. The old saying that a little knowledge is a dangerous thing is quite apt for this phase of my life.

There were times when I questioned my ability to continue, when thoughts of suicide were prevalent, when a longing for release was all I could think about. Introspection and the group discussions helped greatly when this happened. Although feeling very bad about myself I could recall and use the contents of the course to my benefit, even if they didn't feel helpful at the time.

Despair at ever leading a *normal* life was high. I longed for the way I had been. All the time, however, I hid this, sometimes from myself, dismissing it as a fantasy, putting on my public face and adopting a personality that was, outwardly, confident and calm. This, generally, cost me dearly when I reached the sanctuary of my apartment. The self doubts and recriminations would flood over me, driving back down, allowing *The Beast* to roam at will.

It was now into late October, five months since I had made the suicide attempt, and I was dreading the Christmas period. I had worked every Christmas for many years and the thought of being alone with only the TV and the re runs of movies was beginning to concern me. Would I be able to handle my thoughts, would the time of year beat me down? I knew that these kinds of thoughts would probably lessen the likelihood of a serious dip in my behavior. Still I was not looking forward to the holiday season. I hoped that this year the Zulus might win the battle of Rourke's Drift, that more prisoners would escape during the Great Escape, that outdated and

A Cheerful Depression

overly sentimental Christmas movies would be replaced with high octane action films. Of course, this was not to be the case. We have to indulge our sentimentality with this annual ritual of sloppy mush.

I made no special plans for the holidays. I would follow my normal daily routine. If there was something worth while watching on the television, I would watch it. I contemplated attending midnight mass and dismissed it because it would mean staying up too late, breaking my routine. In reality, it was thought of a busy church, having to be in close proximity to others, have to don the public persona. No, I decided I would be better off on my own. Talking of Christmas, I have noticed that one of the pubs in town started advertising its Christmas lunches in April this year. Is this not ridiculous. How much earlier are they going to start reminding us that the year is about to end? Will the shops now start their campaign in August, snow covered cottages and icy chocolates being displayed at the warmest time of the year? I truly believe we have, as a society lost the concept of festivals like Christmas. It appears to have become a time when the predominant feelings are greed and jealousy. A time to beat the Jones' at their own game. With the opening hours of the shops there is no feeling of a holiday. It never ceases to amaze me how shoppers pile up their trolleys with days worth of shopping, day after day in the build up to a holiday. Yet the shops are only closed for one day over Christmas. All that waste, all that effort for one day. It seems illogical. Christmas should be time for celebrating, for children to enjoy their presents. Not for gluttony and an excess of alcohol. Any why bother having family and friends over to lunch, when last year and the year before arguments ensued? What is the point of courting disaster year after year?

Yes, I was, I decided, quite happy to be on my own. I could feel miserable, or not, depending entirely on my thoughts, and not have to rely on others to drag me down.

I make no apology for my thoughts with regard to religious festivals. I am sure that there are many who agree with me. I am just so very tired of the hypocrisy that surrounds us on a daily basis. And it's not just the hypocrisy towards others; it's hypocrisy to one's self. The self delusion that perfection is exuded from each pore of the body, that only goodness and light is offered to others is, at times so transparent, it is sickening to observe. I am convinced these hypocrites believe they fart eau d'cologne.

Are these thoughts a product of the illness, has the illness contributed in some way? No, at least, I don't think so. It is true that hypocrisy is seen in others when they have to deal with their perception of mental ill health. The aversion to the person who is ill, in much the same way as some individuals find it difficult to deal with physical disability. But it is also due to the fact that I have seen changes, over the last fifty eight years, in values, honesty and integrity. There appears to be a lot less of these values displayed overtly in this present age. Politicians and police chiefs are always going on about the lack of respect to others and property, that is displayed by the younger generation. However, the younger generation displays no respect for themselves. They have no respect for their bodies and minds, the over indulgence in alcohol and drugs is but one example of this. And who do they learn this behavior from, their parents and grandparents. It could, I suppose, be argued that the evolution of ever more rigorous Health and Safety requirements has resulted in the molly coddling of a whole generation, in an expectancy that, should something go wrong, there is always someone to blame. There is no sense of standing on one's own two feet and accepting responsibility for one's actions, or the actions of the children. Should a child become an alcoholic at the age of fifteen, it is not their fault. It is the fault of legislation which permits the sale of alcohol, the fault of the shops and pubs that have special offers. Never their own fault, they are to be pitied and looked after. Now I do not have a problem with treatment of these children, or adults. I do have a problem in that it is not recognized that it is on their shoulders. Has the word NO disappeared from the English language? Has the responsibility of taking control of our own destinies been taken away from us by a nanny state?

I often feel that I am responsible for my illness, that somehow I brought this on myself. I have only recently recognized that this is an unfair verdict. Yes, I have lived the life I chose, I, and only I, made the decisions which affected me. But no, the illness was not my fault.

It was during the deep and meaningful discussion with the ever optimistic Samuel. God he could be hard work with his cheery, positive attitude. Sorry Samuel, I'm being just a tad facetious here. That said he did, however, achieve the desired effect, making me more positive about myself. It was the meaning of the term Post-traumatic Stress Disorder. As I have previously said I thought it unthinkable that I could be suffering from this, after all it was more associated with war veterans, guys returning from Iraq and Afghanistan. Wearing his bright orange shirt, Samuel explained, most patiently, that Combat Stress and PTSD were different. PTSD was associated more with events seen or experienced rather than being in an active combat situation. This could be one event or several which built up for a long period. A car accident, an assault, bereavement being only a few.

I have seen my share of dead bodies, the jumper outside the hotel in Edinburgh being the last, a visit to a morgue to witness an autopsy at the age of eighteen being the first. I have even assisted in performing CPR on a guest who had a heart attack, while waiting for the ambulance. He survived, despite our ministrations. Prior to the jumper the last corpse I saw was one of my employees. We had working on a theft ring in conjunction with police and he was performing his normal duties when he was shot, five times in the back and then, when he didn't go down, twice in the back of the head.

We will never know if it was because of his involvement in the investigation or if he was in the wrong place at the wrong time, a victim of a senseless crime. However, I remember that as he was lying there, with the Forensic people sticking their fingers and probes into his head wounds, I was casually talking to a rather attractive police woman. I believe that, at that time and place, we had all become inured to violent death. Around that particular shopping center, the security for which was the responsibility of my company, there had been in the region of eleven violent deaths in two months, seven from gunshots and four from knives. I do remember thinking that I was becoming callous, too hardened to it all. I had to deal with the family, make arrangements to ensure their financial stability, in this fortunately we had a more adequate employee insurance scheme for just such an eventuality.

I suppose there are also instances where I might have ended up as a corpse lying on a road or sidewalk. In one case I had been visiting this same shopping center at night. This was a regular occurrence and I never carried a firearm on these visits. Anyhow, there was group of drunken men gathered outside one of the exits. My staff member was having difficulty controlling them and I intervened, talking to the group while I sent him for assistance. Things took a turn for the worse and I felt that it was going to get out of hand. Now I was confronted with a group of nine well, built males, with the possibility that some of them could be armed in some way. I pulled the one who seemed to be the leader in front of me and backed against a small wall. My thought was that I had to buy some time until my guys could get there. To secure him I put him in a head hold and informed his friends that any movement and I would break his neck. We stood like that for what felt like an eternity; it was only a matter of a couple of minutes. My point is that these types of confrontation were the norm, not only for me, but for my employees and,

A Cheerful Depression

obviously the police.

Another case was when a smaller group of four thought they would mug me, three distracting me while the fourth tried to rip off my hip pocket to gain access to my wallet. This time I managed to pull two of them with me between two parked cars. To this day I remember the coherent thought that I should strike out, which I did. At this resistance they quit and fled the scene. I retained my wallet and my trousers, thankfully remained intact. Well worth the money paid for quality clothing.

Another time I was not so lucky, I did not have any place to go to in order to reduce the odds. It was in middle of the town square and I had just left the bank. Now these guys must have thought that I had drawn money and decided to relieve me of it. I hadn't but they couldn't know that. I dealt with the three in front of me but was unaware of a fourth who had come up behind me. He must have thought that my internal organs were in need of servicing or tuning as he proceeded to stick a Phillips screwdriver in the left side of my back. I disposed of him and, fortunately, in doing so he left the screwdriver sticking in me. Why fortunately? Well it may have damaged an organ and it required an x ray prior to the removal. It didn't make a big hole and there was the minimal amount of blood but a good shirt was bloody ruined.

All the above took place within six months of each other. I want to stress that I was not alone being a victim of crime. I will give an example. A busy Saturday morning in the center of town and a woman had drawn cash from an ATM. A man was behind, shot her in the back of the head and took her money. Senseless and impossible to predict.

Did any of the above contribute to the PTSD as part of the depression?

The consensus is that they did contribute. A sustained involvement in this type of activity over my life must have had an effect. I hear the question – why did I do it? Well, I could have avoided it. However, I believed that a good manager should be able to perform any task required of his employees, to lead from the front. It would have been taken as weakness not to be as good as, if not better, than anyone I employed. I suppose I have been lucky in these escapades, there may have been a bit of skill involved but it mostly comes down to luck, bred through a high level of self-confidence in my abilities to deal with most situations. There also seems to have been bad luck, in that I was always walking into these situations, a classic case of being in the wrong place at the wrong time.

The reason I recount the above is to demonstrate the kind of life I, and many others like me, led in the Security industry. I would not presume for a moment that I am alone in suffering PTSD. It was a violent society in which we lived. If you will bear with me I will try to describe some of aspects of daily life for everyone at that time.

It was the period between the release of Nelson Mandela and his election to President. While there was euphoria there were also still high levels of poverty which resulted in a shocking crime rate. People lived in houses surrounded by high walls topped with razor wire, burglar bars covered windows and a security gate protected the door. The more affluent had sophisticated alarm systems outside and inside their homes, motion detectors on the walls and even a gate house with a 24/7 security guard. A return home from work was, effectively, a return to a comfortable prison, the bars were more ornate, and the surrounding more comfortable, but still a self-imposed prison. Car jacking was rife. Car windows were kept closed and doors locked. Everyone was conscious of their personal security. Even passive submission to a robbery was not any guarantee of escaping an attack, even death. The

A Cheerful Depression

lives of ordinary working people, black and white were blighted by this crime. It was often the case that the black person was targeted to a greater extent. A criminal will, after all, target the weak and defenseless. To think of the number of undiagnosed people still walking around having been the victim of crime is frightening.

But it was my job and I didn't think twice about it. I slept well at night and never felt threatened or insecure. It was a fact of life. I sometimes wonder if the return to the UK and the relative safety and secure environment in some way brought the PTSD to the fore. I am told that it was more than likely as a by product of the anxiety and depression. I do know that the loss of the self-confidence is one of the hardest things to deal with, the feeling that I am no longer in control. It is a loss of a large part of my personality and I sorely miss it. I know the self-confidence will return, the self esteem, possibly not to the extent as before, but then I don't need those abilities anymore.

Of course, here I have to stress that most of the population lived in some comfort and safety, although aware of the overall situation and the necessary measures to keep safe.

During this time I lived on my own, what woman in their right mind would want to be associated with a job like mine? I had been divorced from the last wife for three years and enjoyed the experience of only having myself to look after. A young feller who I hired as my Operations Manager did get married, happily, and performed his job very well. I did not ask of him the same I asked of myself. I suppose I wanted to protect him to a certain degree. Not that he wasn't competent and able to cope with most things, he was. It just wasn't necessary to put him in the same situations.

To be honest I don't know how his wife coped with the ridiculous hours we worked. He would never shirk away from putting in some extra time. He often told me that he would cover for me, that it wasn't necessary for me to be there and that I should relax more. I did avail myself of this offer, although staying in the vicinity, available if he required some assistance. I suppose I was guilty of protecting him to a certain extent, but I know I would never have forgiven myself if anything had happened to him. Taking this kind of responsibility is yet another factor in the build up to depression. It doesn't do anyone any good to assume responsibility for events that may be totally outside their control.

I don't know why none of the night terrors involved any of these events. They were unrelated to any specific incident; they were random, maybe influenced by a programme on TV or the contents of a book. The night terrors have largely abated now, when they do return they are just as bad and vivid. One comfort is that they can be explained and it is easier to relax after them. Sleep is even possible. A big relief, a good night's sleep is important to recovery. I would not wish these terrors on my worst enemy, or my ex-wife, they were so bad.

As Christmas approached I now knew a bit more about depression and anxiety. I tried to challenge my thinking when it was beginning to drag me down. I knew what was happening as I started to feel weepy or low. I made every effort to keep positive and push the negative thoughts away. I went out and endured Christmas shopping crowds, telling myself that no one knew what was wrong with me, they couldn't see the torment through the public persona which I now wore as a second skin. If I met someone I knew I would smile and converse with them, disguising the facts of my illness.

To this day, despite knowing what I know now, I still have a tendency to look at the illness as a stigma, not to be talked about. It is an illogical action, but I, and others, still persist in

A Cheerful Depression

this behavior. Samuel once told me to do things I wanted to do, not what I thought I had to do, *should do*, this makes it easier he told me. Well, it's true, to want to go out, is easier than forcing yourself to it. It's part of the process of removing pressure on yourself to perform. It does get easier, the longer you survive the day to day to process, the easier it becomes.

Liken it, if you will, to the man who threw himself off a tall building. It is recorded that he was heard to say, as he passed each floor, *"so far so good, so far so good"*. This was how I viewed each day.

Extract from journal:

Really slept late, first woke about 07h30, then woken by phone at 08h40, the exercise of yesterday seems to have knocked me out. It worked though, not a bad morning although a bit lethargic. Went out for a walk later on but still feeling unloved, unwanted. Don't know why I care, I don't need anyone, they all wear two faces anyway and are hypocritical saying what is correct and then hiding if it does not suit their own self interests or fear/comfort levels. It's all a load of bollocks really, I've never noticed meeting too many people like this before, and they all seem to be paranoid and scared of their own shadows. Anyway went for a walk and felt a bit better physically really have not been doing too much over the weekend.

CHAPTER 7

Having started the process of group therapy you would think that the next group would be easier to deal with. Not the case. The same anxieties resurfaced, the same feelings of worthlessness. The next group was to deal with building self esteem. Nothing too threatening there.

The facilitators for this group were Lizelle and Mary. Vivacious and bubbly, Lizelle with a wicked sense of humor with an infectious laugh, Mary the quieter, more reflective of the two. They provided the right balance, complimenting each other's personalities. Making all of us feel at ease and safe from the get go. They were good choices to take us through the process of pointing us in the right direction of regaining some vestige of self esteem.

I have mentioned before the preferred manner of my death and Lizelle, and Lindsay, who was to take a later group, would be my definitive choices for the women. Aside from their marvelous personalities they are both attractive women in their mid thirties, I hope I'm correct in that guess at their ages, it's not something I'm very good at, and they will forgive me if it is erroneous. However, that will have to remain a day dream as they are both happily married. Not to mention the fact that there is a twenty year age gap. I wonder if they like whiskey? Ah, it's a nice thought!

This was a smaller group and I was again the only man. I found myself adopting the role of the male, an instinctive reaction, I suppose, putting on the public persona. The subject matter was as emotive as the anxiety aspect. But again it was interesting to hear another's perspective on the same feelings.

There can be no doubt that self esteem can make us feel good about ourselves and that low self esteem can make us feel

A Cheerful Depression

terrible. It is the confidence in our ability to think, feel and act when facing basic decisions throughout life. It is about respecting yourself, recognizing our own dignity and value as a human being. About being aware and comfortable with our strengths and weaknesses without needlessly criticizing ourselves and trusting ourselves to be able to cope and behave in a consistent manner despite changes occurring around us. Also the belief that we can achieve our personal goals, wants and needs.

A recurring theme throughout the six weeks was the difficulty each of us had with the *NO* word. We thought it to be an expression of selfishness. This is certainly a negative connotation. Yes it can be selfish to put yourself first if you are ignoring the needs of others. However, a philosophy of enlightened self interest in ourselves, or being interested in ourselves as well as others, is desirable. Sometimes it may be necessary to be selfish to ensure there is a balance between our own needs and those of others.

The skill of looking after ourselves and paying attention to our needs is an important one. It involves being assertive enough to say *"this is what I like", "this is what I need"*. To treat ourselves by doing things we enjoy. Some people, myself included, have never learned to look after themselves in this way; they feel guilty and view it as being selfish.

Here we come back to that vicious cycle of negative thoughts and behavior. Negative expectations which limit behavior. I was particularly bad at this, always expecting the worst, continually stuck in a pessimistic outlook, viewing everything as a worst case scenario; sure that nothing would ever go right for me.

The most obvious ways in which this is reflected is our attitude and behavior towards others. Even friends can be pushed away while dealing with strangers leaves you quaking in your boots. Isolation and withdrawal is seen as the safest method of dealing with these thoughts. True it is the safest option, but we cannot live our lives behind a wall albeit a mental one, believing it protects us from the world outside. I don't think you have to be suffering from depression to feel like this some of the time. When things become too much it can be good to retreat and take time to yourself. It is when it affects our every day lives that it becomes more of a concern. I am sure that we are all familiar with acrophobia, the fear of going out. It is very easy to fall into this. One day of hiding leads to another and yet another, days flow into weeks and all of a sudden the fear of going out is astronomical. A self-imposed prison sentence. The panic experienced is real and terrifying, it feeds upon itself. Can this really be related to self esteem – absolutely. I know my thoughts were, if I cannot like myself, how others could possibly like me. I had literally hated and loathed myself since my suicide attempt. I refused to believe that others could feel anything other than contempt for me.

For me a horrible thought rose to the surface, a great white shark swimming up from the depths, to attack and maim me. It was the belief that I would never again find someone to hold and to hold me. To love and be loved became a want, a desire which consumed me. I was convinced that I would never again have this experience and, to this date, I have not found that person. My own fault as I have never placed myself in a situation where it could happen. My fear, stemming from the poor self esteem and lack of self-confidence, the knowledge that no sensible person would find me attractive, driving all logic and rational thought from my mind. The fear of rejection, possibly, the fear of showing my weaknesses, probably. I hope that one day I will have conquered this and that love will come my way again. I was not alone in this. As the others were in relationships at that time they did not have this fear to the extent that I had. There was, however, insecurity in their relationships, doubts that

A Cheerful Depression

arose with regard to the ability to maintain it. I could compare these doubts generated in the mind to the heads of Medusa. Each being a separate entity, competing with the other for dominance, pulling each individual in different directions, vying for prominence.

Being deeply loved by someone
gives you strength;
while loving someone deeply
gives you courage.

That is a quote from Lao Tzu of which I am fond. I have loved deeply. I have lost that love. That is incorrect, I never lost the love, I lost the person I loved. Hopefully love remains no matter what happens as painful as that can be, time does dull the pain and leaves pleasant memories of happier times. Of course, this can be a double edged sword. Comparisons are inevitably made with the memory and the result is always the same, nothing compares favorably. I suppose it part of human nature to do this; if it is not then I am sicker than we thought. The depression must have an adverse affect on this, making the memory more poignant and the differences keener. I have felt deep hurt, emptiness and pain as a result of that loss. It was a love that never ran its course; it was abruptly and tragically terminated. I can attest to the fact that such a love can give you strength. The strength to protect, to overcome all obstacles. The courage it gives is a thing of wonder. Courage to feel, to state your feelings, to commit and to love freely, with no restrictions placed upon the giving of your love. I never found again that kind of love over the last thirty years. I have believed myself to be in love, I have committed to a relationship, I have tried to make myself open and honest in those relationships but I have never felt that strength of love.

I don't know if I ever will, but I'm willing to try. I don't envy the woman with whom I try. She is competing with a memory. Nothing can eradicate that memory. Perhaps, I do not want to eradicate that memory. It has not dimmed with time which is possibly why this quote is so relevant.

Time is the fire in which we burn
Delmore Schwartz

I can, with certainty, tell you that I have cared very deeply for everyone I have been in a relationship with, I have not wanted to hurt them, upset them.

Love is only a four letter word. Yet it encompasses all the other adjectives we use to describe our feelings. Happiness, hope, affection, caring, fear to name but a few. Undoubtedly there is a chemical in the brain which is released when we feel a combination of all these emotions. It is the only word we have in the English language which covers all the bases, and it is misused in so many contexts. I believe that, if you asked one hundred people their definition of love there would be one hundred differing answers. It is an intangible feeling we all long for but is as elusive as the pot of gold at the bottom of a rainbow. I have, during this period, doubted my ability to love. A string of failed relationships attest to that, in my mind. I don't know if I have remained in a relationship as a matter of habit. I think that a lot of partnerships are like that. People fall into the habit of being together, the comfort of routine, and reach the stage where they cannot imagine life without the other. I am not going to debate whether this is right or wrong. If it works and it makes them happy then why not? But that leads us to the happy word. I believe that happiness is perceived, that, in a relationship it is the normal state of affairs which make us happy. The personalities of the partners become meshed and the happiness is derived from the fact that there is a constant. This can be the quality of life which we all strive for, watching and appreciating the achievements of family members as they grow older. However, I do not believe happiness is easily gained; it takes work and respect for others. I do not think that money or material possessions provide this happiness. Although, I must admit, I would love to try that method. I have been envious of this kind of sustained love and happiness. I said as much in my suicide note. Nevertheless I have been unable to attain this in thirty years and this is where the doubt comes in. If I was not able to achieve this when I was younger, how on earth am I going to even come close now? These feeling drive my mood down.

Can this be resolved? Popular fiction has us believe that there is someone out there for everyone and we will meet them, given time. My doubts are explained away as part of the low self esteem and loss of self-confidence which will work itself out, given time. But I have to ask myself if that is the case. Will the fear of a relapse into the darker days happen at some stage? What if I have been lucky enough to find someone special and this happens? Personally I do not know if I will be able to cope with a relapse, I do not know if I have the strength, or the will, to go through this whole process again. And what of the other person? Would they be able to cope with it? Would I have the common sense to tell them about my feelings without the fear of driving them away? Some of you will say that is what love is all about. Accepting each other as you are, no matter what. I would like to think that my fears and concerns are irrational and that I will not have a relapse. That with my new found introspective attitude and knowledge about my inner self; I will be a better person as a result of this illness.

That, however, raises yet another question – is too much introspection a good thing? How do we gauge? Is it possible that too much thinking and analyzing the thought process can, in itself, become destructive? The answer to these questions will become clearer as time goes on and the recovery is complete. I have to believe that the recovery will be total and there will be no relapse. Also I have to believe that, as my mind returns to normality, the amount of time spent on these concerns will lessen as I re learn to accept the workings of my mind on a less distorted level.

I will be honest and state that I would still like to meet someone. That, if it does happen, I can push the memory to its proper place and accept and give an unconditional love. I am sure this desire is a by product of the depression, that my low opinion of myself clouds reasonable thinking on these lines. I certainly and fervently hope this to be the case. This, to some, may reek of self pity and, if I'm honest, it may very well be the case. However, I use it to demonstrate the distorted thinking which becomes prevalent with depression.

Having said all that I do not believe that I have lost the capacity to care, and care deeply about others. There are occasions when this caring has helped to take my mind off my own feelings and try, in whatever small way, to be of help. This can take the form of just being an ear, someone to bounce ideas off, to express their feeling which, in turn, helps them to find a solution. There have been times when I have felt disgust at my illness, thinking it not as bad as some of the things I was hearing. As they say, complaining about a sore toe is put into perspective when you meet a person without a leg. I have never found anyone, though, obvious exceptions here, who could understand what I was experiencing. They will listen attentively but you know that the understanding is missing. Depression is an illness that can be difficult for someone outside to grasp. It is too complex to explain fully. That is probably why I am trying to write it all down. As you can see, even up to this point alone, it would have taken hours and hours of talking to cover the points I have mentioned so far.

It is entirely plausible that the loneliness of a depressive illness has brought on these feelings of wanting a companion to hold. Perhaps it's the necessity to be held, to return to the mother's breast and be comforted. I do not know if I adopt the fetal position when I sleep, but would be surprised if I did. It

A Cheerful Depression

is, after all a seeking of comfort, the security of the womb.

Taking these thoughts further, another question has entered my thinking. It is not a constructive one and can be viewed as part of the overall distortion. In a world with controlled births would I have received a vasectomy on reaching puberty and would I have been banned from marriage, restricted to occasional and fleeting relationships with prescribed women? It may not have been a bad thing, had this world existed. It would certainly have saved both others and me from a world of hurt. I do not believe, no, I know, I have been a good father. I have always liked moving around too much and children were cumbersome in this process. In conjunction with ex wives, I made decisions which, at the time appeared reasonable, but were wrong. Unfortunately the clock cannot be turned back and mistakes corrected. How I wish it was possible.

I would like to think that this thought process is not the same as the prevalent thinking among the younger generation who seem to think they have to be in a relationship continuously from puberty onwards. It appears to me that they cling to one person to the exclusion of all others, limiting themselves and their experiences by doing so. I constantly see the possessive nature of this, mainly in boys. They should be playing the field. I think it is wrong to try and develop a meaningful relationship in the teenage years. I know I didn't, and I enjoyed every minute with every girl.

This kind of thinking, to conform, is, I believe, damaging. How can they ever learn to be happy with themselves, comfortable on their own and learn to cope on their own, if they are constantly seeking out another person. Watching, there often appears to be desperation in the search for a new person. To me that indicates that there wasn't much substance in the first place. The expectation also seems to be that, instead of seeing each other at school, or for the occasional date at weekends, that they become joined at the hip from day one.

I do not know the scientific thinking on this amount of reliance, but it is my opinion that it cannot be good for anyone, never mind the young. It must have some affect on their development. Again, in the interest of fairness, I am sure that there are many youngsters who do not fall into this category. It is merely an observation I make after having dealt with and worked alongside many youngsters.

My way of thinking could be criticized for promoting promiscuity among the young. Not at all. I do not believe that sex should be entered into lightly. I think the world would be a better place, especially in the light of the increase of Sexually Transmitted Diseases, if both boys and girls held back on the actual sex act until far later in life. This may also help in the relationship stakes. It would develop as friendship as opposed to sex. Possibly that is why they cling to each other, a dependency on the other for sex. I have always believed that sex is a by product of a relationship, an essential way to communicate the feelings about each other, the passion that only two people who have respect and love for the other can feel. I find that to use the term, to make love to someone is more meaningful and true, for me anyway, than the act of having sex with someone. To have sex implies an impersonal act. To make love depicts meaning and caring for the other person.

You see the repeating, self destructive pattern that emerges. The taking on yourself the blame for all the wrongs in the past, completely ignoring the possibility that not all was your fault. That other people, or circumstances, may have contributed. That is the whole point of these sessions. To try and convert, to turn around, this cycle of distorted thinking. After all memories and experiences are what makes us what we are today. They are to be cherished and brought out to

A Cheerful Depression

look on with fondness. We should not permit regrets brought on by these recollections to become the overriding factor. It is natural to regret some aspects of the past; it is not natural to allow them to overwhelm the good.

An important part of good self-esteem is self-reliance, the ability to enjoy your own company. As I've said already I have always been comfortable with myself, happy to be on my own, not being lonely when I'm alone. I've never really *needed* anyone. It may be viewed as strange that I suffer from such a lack of self esteem if this is the case. The only answer I can think of is that it has become such a habit, normality for me that it is hard to imagine it any other way. Even in the darkest of days I had to be self reliant. There was no other way I could survive on a day to day basis. There was also, I believe, a stubborn pride that made asking for help difficult, if not impossible, at times. It was very much a case of deciding each night what was required the next day and then doing it, no matter the effort or cost as far as anxiety attacks, or what others thought. In retrospect I can see that this was a good thing. It didn't permit me the luxury of hiding away for days at a time. I am glad that I didn't weaken in my resolve to look out for myself, to ask for help in the mundane tasks. These old habits can be wearisome at times. In particular my habit of retiring to bed at the same time of 22h00 every night and then rising at 05h30 can be frustrating. It can make for a long day. What sane person stands up at 05h30 when they can stay in bed until 08h00?

This routine, the adherence to a work schedule became very important to me. Perhaps it was mildly obsessive compulsive, in that it has to be followed. A deviation means an irritable me, uncomfortable as I can only get angry at myself, there is no one else to blame for my sloth. It does mean that all the chores are out of the way early, but that's about the only good thing. I have also controlled the urge to sit and fester in front of the television all day.

I have tried hard to maintain a high level of personal pride. I often feel that I have failed in this, miserably, at times. In one instance I had a photograph taken with Alex McLeish, he was Scotland's football manager at the time, and, when I saw it, I hated it. The way I looked. I thought my smile was horrible. What did do? Firstly I grew a mustache to try and conceal my smile and have ended up with a full beard. I do not know if this has been effective in improving my appearance, in my own opinion. But it does hide the smile which I didn't like. It is also effective in straining coffee and soup, although a nuisance when I have a cold! I have found it funny that the smallest thing can upset me in this regard. My self esteem has sunk to lows where I am not comfortable with anything about myself. This, I have found, is hard to deal with, as no matter what I do to try and make myself presentable, I seem to fall short of the desired result. This makes getting ready to go a long and, sometimes, wearisome process. I notice every crease and crinkle in shirts and trousers, how my shoes are not as shiny as they should be, I stand in front of the mirror and criticize myself, even though there is nothing more I could possibly, with the exception of major plastic surgery. I suppose even then I would find something wrong. I will not contemplate that until I am better and then, with a return of self-confidence I will no longer need it, maybe just maybe.

The constant message from the hospital is always to keep active, mentally and physically. Rising early is my way of achieving these goals. Yes it is cheating to the extent that it permits me to avoid crowds, but I am achieving the goals I have set the previous night. That in itself, deserves a bar of chocolate, I feel. Remember, chocolate is good for you!

Deciding to plan activities which you find enjoyable is a good plan, they said. However, activities which were enjoyable, may not be the same. I used to, for example, enjoy going to the pub for a chat with friends. I do not enjoy that anymore. Good for my health, but hell on conversation. I find it hard to

A Cheerful Depression

debate a point with myself in front of the mirror. I always win, I'm always right. Boring.

The thing with depression is the feeling that there is no meaning, direction, significance or purpose in anything attempted. I often thought to myself first thing in the morning - "what's the point in getting up, what's the point in shaving. No one's going to see me or care." There is no way forward, past the darkness, nothing to help us through the night. Failure in achieving goals results in stress and tension, a lack of control, driving you down.

Thus the goals set have to be achievable, small to begin with, with the object of personal values and belief paramount. If the goal is attainable the work towards it can increase motivation and the release of energy to complete the task.

*"Plan for your future because that is where
you are going to spend the rest of your life"*
Mark Twain

I have set myself goals insofar as this writing is concerned. I strive to attain the daily goals in the time spent in front of my computer. I have a goal with regard to the length of this book and the timeframe for completion. I do fail in these goals, particularly on a daily basis. I inevitably feel guilty when this happens and resolve to double my efforts the next day. If writing this achieves nothing else, it has given me the motivation to push ahead. I will admit that, when I do fail to reach a daily goal, I always try to rationalize it to myself, to make excuses for the failure. I was getting a sore back, I was cold, I was hungry or I had to go out to the shops or for a walk. I believe the difference now is the fact that I know what I am doing when I make these excuses. It doesn't ease the guilt over the failing, but I am beginning to understand myself and accept my failings.

What I have been doing in making these excuses is procrastinating. It is easy to do. By doing so I avoid frustration and anxiety. We all procrastinate; we put off mowing the lawn to watch a football game. We delay writing a presentation for work, leaving it till the last minute. Personally I have always found this to be the best way. I liked the pressure of having a tight deadline to work to and it always worked out well. Now the only deadlines I have are those set by me, but they are just as compelling. However, I have found that even completion of a small part of a task makes me feel better than avoiding it altogether. It is still a success, an achievement.

I sometimes ask myself if I am a perfectionist. I would never have considered that to be the case, but this train of thought has been somewhat forced upon me. A perfectionist is someone who keeps emotions under tight control and has a fear of showing vulnerability, of losing control. I guess you can recognize me in that description. Behind perfectionism, it is believed, lurk deep unrecognized fears and needs. The perfectionist is motivated by fear of failure. In failing to reach a goal he feels a failure as a person. He is never satisfied by achievements, needing to constantly strive for more and more. It is a difficulty in letting things go and varying standards according to time and effort needed. Perfection is an unattainable illusion guaranteed to make us feel like failures and thus make us more vulnerable to depression. When I look at this I think of the desire to love and have to ask if my perception of love is the same kind of illusion, something that is never attainable. These are hard questions to answer. Harder to ask of yourself, to face the truth.

The way I have tried to deal with this is by lowering my standards, by deliberately limiting the time spent on a task. Instead of telling myself that I will spend eight hours on the computer, I will say that I will spend time on the computer today. If I achieve 80% of what I think I would normally have

A Cheerful Depression

achieved then I am happy.

I also try to enjoy recounting my experiences here and try to ignore the final word, the finished product and what that will entail. I will finish when I finish. Then and only then I will deal with what follows. Needless to say this does not always work, but that it is not a product of the illness. We all think about the future, tomorrow or a year from now, and I am no different. I know I think about the time when I won't feel like this anymore. I plan how I will get there. I have not set any goals to achieve this normality. I know that it is totally impracticable and unrealistic. I settle for the daily goals and savor every achievement.

As much as I hate to admit it, I think that I may have been striving for perfection prior to this. I think, in particular, of a thesis I had to submit for my Honours. I worked at it for ages, constantly changed, revising, adding and removing parts until I had to submit it. I was sure that it was useless and would be thrown out of the window, that it was incomplete. It wasn't.

I would have achieved the same result, in all likelihood, if I had finished it, corrected it and left it, content that it was the best I could do. It would also have saved me a lot of worry and stress, prior to the interview and an explanation of my theories.

Here I would like to make an assumption. And that is that you've seen the breakdown of the word assume – to assume is to make an *ASS* of *U* and *ME.* I mention this because when upsetting circumstances occurred automatic thoughts ran through my mind, distorted, negative thoughts. I assumed the worst without any testing of the evidence. I would think I *should* be able to do something because I had always been able to do it, and make myself frustrated and angry. I made all the wrong assumptions. I was trying to do something because I thought I should do it not because I wanted to do it.

Now I make a conscious effort to avoid using the "should" word. I ask could I do that. I rarely do something because I "must". Obviously all of this is not something that happens quickly, it has taken a long time to adopt this way of thinking and I'm not out of the woods yet. It is not yet an automatic process and I catch myself returning to the negative ways all the time. But again, the process has a beginning, the end is inconsequential, it will come in time. Wouldn't it be nice if the world was a fair and reasonable place? That will, unfortunately, never happen. It's said that bad things happen to good people. Sometimes its random, sometimes it's because of the unreasonableness of others and sometimes because of our own imperfections. To expect others to treat us fairly, when they often have their own ideas about what is fair, is to invite disappointment. I have, during the really bad times, and even now, often asked, *"why me?", "what have I done to deserve this?"* We are all guilty of imploring God when things are bad and, for this reason, I sometimes expect a dark cloud to form over my head, parting to allow a hand with a finger pointing directly at me and a deep voice booming, *"Because I Don't Like You".* That may be a worst case scenario, but it would be definitive proof that there was a God and he knew what was happening, was in control. That's a positive thought, although it could be described as distorted thinking, particularly by the Church.

One distorted thought that is not fair is to label yourself. I have called myself a loser, a failure, useless and many more names. This we were told is pointless, a human being is too complex to be described by one word. If you do something stupid, don't call yourself stupid; rather tell yourself that it was a silly thing to do, stupid sometimes, but not always. It is hard to accept that being fallible is an everyday part of life. By giving yourself a negative label makes it harder to accept a compliment on something well done. In doing this you are rejecting, or discounting, the fact that you have worked long and effectively. If you do this you are negating the

A Cheerful Depression

accomplishment – they are no longer fun. I found that I was quite happy to compliment others, bad at accepting compliments.

Why could I give credit when it was due and not do myself the same favour? Simple, I didn't feel I had done anything to my credit. I often ask myself why I would like positive comments to be made about me, but, when they come I never believe them. I prefer to think the person is lying merely to boost my self esteem and does not mean what they say. There is never even a moment's consideration that what they are saying may be true. What, I wonder, will make me happy again? If I knew the answer to that I would be able to resolve all these issues. During the course of this illness I know that something like winning the lottery would not make me happy, it might bring a bit of joy, but I know it would be short lived. It would probably produce more anxiety than anything. One thing I do know, is that I would certainly like to try and cope with that anxiety.

It comes down to separating unpleasant external situations without condemning the core self, trying to deal with it with a realistic, upbeat and immediate response. A response that reinforces the self worth, pushing aside the external influences. Admitting you made a mistake but recognizing that you are still a worthwhile person, who has value, whose potential is infinite and unchangeable, is an essential skill to develop if you are to beat low self esteem. Again it's easy to say this, to tell us as a group that it's the right thing to do. It is infinitely harder to do and takes as much practice as a piano virtuoso. To all of us it was another high mountain to be scaled.

I would like to draw a comparison here. There is a mountain in the Rockies, near Lake Louise which has a cable car to take you to the summit. From there you can see north and south, endless mountain peaks. This recovery was the same as looking at those mountains. One after another, stretching endlessly towards the horizon. No sooner is one peak scaled, than there is another filling the distance.

Ego. Now there's a word to play with. Does high self esteem mean that an individual has a high or super ego? I suppose so. I would never like to see myself with the ego akin to a politician. Their egos are super sized and impervious to any criticism. It is, of course, good to have the self belief in decision making and action. But at the exclusion of all else? I would like to think that I have never allowed my ego to interfere with my sense of fairness and of treating everyone with the respect they deserve, no matter what their beliefs. A few politicians have stated that their support decision to go to war was also based in a trust that God, and the CIA, was on their side and that right would prevail. Their egos, however, omitted, precluded the fact that the other side also had a belief system. They also believed that they were conducting a Holy War against the oppression of the Western World. I am not condoning the methods used to further their goals in their Jihad. I am merely making the point that all these super egos, on any side, are what drive us into conflict. I truly believe that this kind of person is out of touch with reality on any practical level, ignoring or, worse, not caring what others think. Think back to the time when Bill Clinton started the trend of using his trousers as ankle warmers, the way he dealt with that was disgraceful. In fairness, who but Americans would hang onto their dirty clothing, not sending it to the dry cleaners for months? Keeping seminal stains as a souvenir?

The most offensive aspect, to me, of this whole ego trip is the fact that it is a case of trying to impose our values and standards on peoples with a different set of standards and values, which have worked for them for thousands of years. It seems to me that this is done with no consideration for these facts, they are either ignored or, far worse, there is an unwillingness to understand and adapt to them. This is not a

A Cheerful Depression

new approach for politicians unfortunately. Take McMillan's "Winds of Change" speech. Winds of change were sweeping through Africa. Too right they were. After that there was the Mau Mau rising in Kenya, the conflict in the Congo, which continues to this day and, of course Zimbabwe. No one took into account the completely different cultures when initiating this.

If we use Zimbabwe as an example. After Ian Smith's Unilateral Declaration of Independence in the late sixties, Britain moved heaven and earth to isolate the country. Rigorous sanctions were imposed. Warships cruised the waters of Mocambique to prevent goods being landed by sea. The result was that the economy flourished. Yes there was a war against the freedom fighters. In perspective, though, it was a war of politics.

The freedom fighters were trained and funded by the Communist states, North Korea being one who was actively involved. The goal of the communists was to gain a foothold in Africa. The goal of America, through the CIA, was to combat this covertly. Politicians on both sides were responsible for a loss of life and, more importantly, the way of life of the indigenous population. Egos of men who had absolutely no understanding of what they were doing, deciding the future and fate of countless people, taking decisions based on the values they held. Egos are responsible for a lot of suffering. In the present day we have a terrible situation in Zimbabwe. Mugabe is increasingly seen as being accountable for genocide and violence. I have to ask if the egos of the politicians are preventing the same kind of action against him as was taken against the Smith government.

However, I suppose, for the rest of us, a mix of good self esteem and moderate levels of ego are the best course. The middle road, where we make an effort to balance our decisions with consideration for others, and for the consequences of our actions. To accept that we can be wrong, it is human nature to err, admit that mistake and try to rectify it. It takes a good person to admit an error of judgment, but it is better to do so than adversely affect the lives of others.

I suppose you could look at the above and say that I have a healthy ego. That may be so but it does not take a lot to have, and express, an opinion against a wrong. Sometimes it is easier to rail against an injustice in this format than it is to actually do something about it. Quite what I could do about it, beyond this, I do not know. One thing is for sure I will not be voting for Brown in the next election. The man has the charisma and jaw movements of a crocodile!

To illustrate the similarity between those of us in this group, I would like to tell you about one of the women. She had been having difficulty in going out and one of the goals she had set herself was to go to the pub at the weekend. She went out and assumed her public face, trying to present the same person she had been before the illness. She was a naturally extrovert person, she had a job which, in my opinion, required a great deal of self esteem and confidence. However, once she was out she read the wrong messages regarding her behavior. She persevered trying to be positive and outgoing. It didn't take long for her to feel inadequate and unwanted. A chance comment, taken the wrong way and that was it. It was the same for all of us, to some degree or the other. We all operated under the illusion that we could see what others were thinking about us. We made assumptions, always wrongly, that bad things were being said or thought about us. This is what makes us want to hide away, drives us to tears of frustration and hurt. The feeling that it is pointless to try and explain what is going on, never mind trying to disguise the fact that we are uncomfortable in any given situation.

The reluctance to go out socially is not confined to this illness. I am sure we have all experienced the feeling that it

A Cheerful Depression

would be better to stay at home, prior to an evening out with friends. This can be because of tiredness, a desire to watch a particular programme on television or just the feeling that it will not be much fun. How often have we found, however, that the evening has been a success and we have enjoyed ourselves? The only difference with us is that we give in to our nagging little voice telling us that it is safer to stay away from these situations, to remain within our own comfort zone. After all, to venture out is return to a state of anxiety and all the associated discomfort.

Depression is an exacerbation of normal responses to everyday situations. Distorted thinking. I found it handy to remind myself of the basics – the sun will set and then rise the next morning. Life, no matter how poor a quality, will go on. If I maintain my schedule I will get things completed.

To start each day as the beginning, yesterday has gone and nothing can be changed. Each day is not a rehearsal or practice for the following one, you only get one shot at it, so go for it, do the best you can, that's all you, or anyone else, can ask of yourself.

CHAPTER 8

The mood swings continued into the New Year. At the time they still seemed as bad as they had ever been. It sometimes felt as if there were three steps forward and four back. The one thing I tried to remember was that they were never as bad as they had been. To dip into a low mood during the course of the day is frustrating and annoying, even more so if you feel you have been quite successful in achieving the aims of the day. This stage of the recovery was hard because of that return to a low mood. What, I think, made it more difficult, was the fact that there could be a period of days, a week, when all was going smoothly and then, for no reason, there was a dip, which could last for days. I found that when I woke in the morning my attitude for the day was already determined. I have managed to successfully turn around a bad start to the day by persevering at the tasks I had set myself. I have not always been able to reach the targets set, but I have completed some of the task, despite myself. I will admit that there are times when I have to redo something I have attempted when feeling down, the upswing in my mood giving me a different perspective. I have now grown accustomed to these mood swings and know that I will snap out of a low mood at some stage, whether it is during the day or when I wake up one morning.

There is a saying that we make our luck. I am undecided on my view of this. It has appeared to me that I have never been lucky. However, that view is dependent of how good luck is perceived. I mean lucky in the manner of good fortune as opposed to surviving the scrapes I have previously described. I have never won a major prize. I have never unexpectedly received a large sum of money or goods. During the course of the last two years, it has seemed as if everything was working against me. Letters would not arrive on time. There appeared to be delay after delay in getting things done. I know this is

A Cheerful Depression

not a matter of luck, rather a fault in the systems. However, it reinforced my feeling that absolutely nothing was going in my favor. I know I used to wake up with the thought that maybe this day would bring some good news in the post. What constitutes good news, I am not sure. The optimistic side of my brain worked overtime. Unfortunately nothing ever arrived. This increased the low moods. Illogical, I know. It was just the feeling that something good was sure to happen to me. This kind of thinking, although positive in a manner of speaking, was as distorted as the other, as destructive in the dashing of hope.

I know that hope is important for every person on the planet. We all have our hopes for a miscellany of things. At the moment my greatest hope is for a full recovery. I hope that this optimistic outlook which can drag me down so quickly, will be justified and that something, anything, which can be described as good will happen. I suppose that one of the difficulties is recognizing that good. I reckon I will have to rely on Samuel to tell me! In addition to failing to recognize it, I worry that it may not make me happy except for a short while. To laugh and smile, even in the face of adversity, as I once used to would be a good thing.

Hope, I believe, is an important aspect of our make up. Everyone has hopes and aspirations; it is what makes the word go round. They obviously differ from person to person. Often it is simply the hope that life circumstances will improve, hope that someone special is waiting around the next corner, hope that career prospects will flourish and personal growth will be rewarding. It can be an intangible something which we pursue endlessly, but which is always there. Without hope we would all end up plodding our way from day to day, mindlessly surviving in a world of pain and woe.

Hope is not something that can be given to us, it is inherent within us. I suppose I am stating the obvious here but it is important to realize that people suffering from depression have no hope that the future holds anything past the misery they are feeling at that time. That is the reason for suicide. There is no hope, no ability to see past that moment in their life when they are at their lowest. Prior to a suicide attempt there is only the realization that it is impossible for things to improve. I believe this applies across the board, in some form. To be without hope is to be in a state of supreme desperation. That feeling of desperation is hard to describe, you are, literally, hopeless, there is no control over your life. Nothing anyone can say will remove that feeling. Talking through the hopelessness is in itself a waste of time – hopeless. If, as in my case, the suicide attempt fails, the sense of hopelessness is increased ten fold. The result is that you can officially describe yourself as hopeless because you failed yet again. After all, you have to be hopeless, useless, if you cannot even manage to take your own life.

It is the same when efforts are made to try and describe the illness to others. It is a hopeless task and you give up. The feeling is the same as the drunk sitting at the bar and telling the barman that his wife doesn't understand him. A person with depression can sit and honestly say that no one understands him. This may reek of self pity but it is true, the knowledge that no one understands is as real to a person with a depressive illness as the sun rising in the morning. This sense of hopelessness can drive you down in an ever increasing spiral, if it is permitted to continue. Fortunately, there is hope inside all of us and it does tend to surface at some point, if we survive the initial fall to rock bottom. The saying of *"where there's life there's hope"* is very relevant and it is a life raft to which we must cling when the waves of hopelessness are dragging us down into the depths of despair.

I know there have been days over the last two years when I have felt overwhelmed. When the despair has reached record levels. As time has gone on, however, that hope has always

A Cheerful Depression

surfaced. Things may not have gone along as I would have liked, but hope has always pulled me back from the brink, long enough, at least, to regain control over my thinking. I do sometimes ask myself if the hope I have on a daily basis is chemically induced by the medication I take in the mornings to assist in improving my mood, after all, I don't really know what I am hoping for, I only know that I will recognize it when I see it, I hope.

The realization that we will never get all we want from life has to temper the hope. That most of the things we decide have an element of risk, because the decisions we make are generally made with a limited amount of information. That, if we make a wrong decision, make a mistake, we can forgive ourselves and accept the fact that we are human.

While in the depths of despair I used to hope that I would be able to regain control over my own destiny. Now I have, I accept responsibility for my actions. I do not believe I can blame any one person for the way my life has turned out. I have re-established the thinking that it is better to face things head on, to accept problems as challenges. I know this is a well used philosophy in business and HR techniques, but it has eluded me for some time now. I can now see again that there is nothing in life that cannot be resolved with a bit of thought and effort. It has taken a long time for me to regain this perspective and I endeavor to maintain it on a daily basis. When it becomes an automatic function again, I will know the end of the recovery is nearing.

Hope, however, can be the Sword of Damocles, double edged and hanging over your head, waiting for a moment of weakness. I have found that there is, at the moment, no happy medium with regard to my hopes. I either soar like an eagle or am down in the Marianas Trench.

To hope, to wish, for something can get out of hand, leading to a horrible disappointment when it does not transpire the way I wanted.

I try hard to temper my hope, my optimism, with a healthy dose of pessimism, a thought that reality is not always what I would like it be, that there will always be disappointments lurking around the corner. I don't know if this optimism is a by product of the medication but I can convince myself that something good is going to happen, believing it and finding excuses as to why it never happened. This feeling is generally at its strongest first thing in the morning, high or low mood is determined the moment I open my eyes. It is really hard to combat and I have, occasionally, become confused at the moment of waking, as to what is real and what is imagined. In much the same way as we all wake from a particularly pleasant dream, wanting to sleep again to recapture it, but being awake and being convinced that the thought in my head is real. Once realization dawns that it is merely a figment of my imagination I find my mood slipping and the negativity returning in full strength.

One of the tools given to me by Samuel was the Emotional Freedom Technique, EFT for short. This is an up and coming therapy with a wide range of applications. It is based on the Meridian system used by the Chinese for thousands of years and is capable of treating mental, emotional and physical problems. It has been gaining in popularity through shows like *Richard and Judy. The Good Morning Show* as well as receiving much positive press in magazines such as *Zest*, *Hello* and even in the *Daily Mail*. It has been described as *"psychological acupuncture"* but without the needles and is quick and easy to learn.

I am not ashamed to say that I was extremely skeptical about this when it was first explained to me. However, I was willing to try anything to help me in my recovery. I don't suppose too many people have heard of this so please bear with me as I

A Cheerful Depression

give a bit of background before going into the principles and method.

EFT was developed in the early 90's by Gary Craig, although it continues to be refined by many people to this day. It is one of the many forms of METs (Median Energy Techniques) now available, and perhaps one of the easiest to learn. It originated from TFT (Thought field Therapy), which was discovered by acupuncturist and psychologist Dr Roger Callahan in the 80's. While Callahan developed the basic concept and structure, Craig had the vision to refine it and make it accessible to everyone. He also, along with many other therapists working in the field, began to realize the broader possibilities for EFT. As a therapeutic technique there is little else to equal its simplicity and effectiveness. Many experienced therapists now report typical success rates of 80-95% for many conditions. Although the immediate history of EFT is short; its future looks to be much longer.

How does it work? Simply put, no one knows for sure. However there are a few theories. It uses the end points of the 12 major meridian channels and the 2 governing vessels found in Chinese medicine. It has been observed that tapping on these points while focusing on the problem, a release takes place clearing the physical or emotional pain being worked on. This has lead to the principle that *"the cause of all negative emotions is a disruption in the body's energy system".* It seems that while experiencing or focusing on a specific problem, and tapping on the meridians that carry the energy, disruptions are cleared and normal function can resume.

When normal function is restored a cognitive shift takes place that can leave the individual wondering what the problem ever was. They then find it hard to believe, and in some cases just don't remember, that they even had the problem. This is known as the Apex effect. This is further heightened by the general disbelief that this technique could ever work. I personally have never experienced this, although I have found it hard to accept that EFT does work.

Another interesting aspect of EFT is that of psychological reversal. This appears to be when the energy flow becomes reversed, although nobody is exactly sure how it works. The outcome is, however, undeniable. Take for example somebody who wants to quit smoking. Anybody familiar with muscle testing would be able to tell you this person should test positive when saying they want to stop. However, most people don't. They still have deeper part of them that wants to carry on smoking. The outcome of this is it is possible to help someone to stop when their will power is not strong enough. In fact it even demonstrates that will power is not best used to overcome addictions. Will power, if used for long durations, is another form of stress on the body. It is great to use in emergency situations, but if used to overcome a craving it is likely that craving will resurface for something else. This is commonly seen when someone stops smoking and starts eating more instead.

There are many other things that EFT can help with, but here I would like to assert that I have used it to combat anxiety, to overcome the fear of going out. It sounds too good to be true. It has, however, helped me lessen anxiety levels, leaving me better able to deal with whatever task I have set myself. I was also extremely self-conscious when I first tried it with Samuel. With his guidance I did manage to concentrate and, surprisingly, found that after three repetitions I felt light headed, a strange sensation of being clearer. This well being did not last, I think I was too skeptical in my approach. However I have persevered and have found it can be helpful. I am not going to try and explain the technique, however, if you want to know more all the information can be found at *www.eft-therapy.com*. Suffice to say that this can be useful in the early stages of anxiety through the more aggressive,

A Cheerful Depression

debilitating stages. You don't even have to be ill to use it. It can be used in the work place to relax or focus the mind. EFT has been shown to be helpful in treating headaches. It is definitely something worthwhile having in your armory for dealing with all aspects of everyday life.

The motto with this must be *"try it on anything"*, although some conditions do have better success rates than others. Many fears and phobias can be removed completely and permanently in just 1 – 2 sessions. Again I have witnessed this first hand when this type of course has been offered at the hotel at a time when I was working. They have brought in pythons which people like me with a fear of snakes have handled after one or two sessions. Again, I have never tried this myself – my fear of snakes is far too great, I believed at the time. However, knowing what I do now, I might be willing to give it a go. If they succeeded in only getting me in the same room as a snake it could be regarded as a resounding success. I wonder if it would work with my fear of relationships!! Of course, this technique is used in conjunction with medical treatment and not as a replacement.

I have never been a big fan of beating myself on or about the head, albeit with only my fingertips, however it was well worth the effort. I suppose, as with most things, I have tried to over analyze this technique while I have been using it. I have not arrived at any conclusions, after all if the experts who devised it do not understand it, who am I to try. However, it may be that the concentration on the act of tapping the various medians and the repetition of the key phrase may take the mind off the problem being addressed. Whatever way you think about it – it does work and is well worth the effort of learning it. There is one example told to me of a nurse at the clinic who was afraid of driving on the motorway.

I do not know the reasons for this, but she was taken through the technique by Samuel prior to driving on the motorway.

She said afterwards that the fear did lessen and she was able to cope with the drive without the fear/nerves that she had, up to that point, always experienced.

I have not tried EFT in respect of friendships, when I'm ready to proceed to that level I may very well try it before I go out. Both to release anxiety and to try and build enough self esteem. I do know that one thing I have yet to do is nurture, and value, friendships. I know I have let things slip badly in this regard. Here I must have hope that I can do this. We all accept friends as part of our lives. It is an unfortunate aspect of this illness, for me, that I have pushed them to all to one side. I have to believe that I have not lost the capacity to rebuild friendships, that I can again accept others for what they are, not for what I want them to be.

So, does hope spring eternal? The unequivocal yes has to be the answer. It certainly keeps me going. I am learning to temper my hopes with rational expectations of both myself and others. A realistic optimism, if you like, to prevent an overreaction of disappointment if things do not my way all the time. I have been like a baby learning to walk and talk, relearning to control my thoughts and understand the various aspects of the illness to effectively combat it. I suppose it could be said that I have had to take my feelings and emotions back to the beginning and learn to understand them all over again. This is particularly true of emotions I have kept buried for most of my life.

One emotion, feeling, is as alien to me as the proper use of the English language is to George Bush, is that of vulnerability. My fervent hope is that this will ease with time. It may be down to the fact that I have opened myself up to a few people. This has been to aid in my recovery and they know all my darkest secrets, desires and fears. Fortunately, they are bound by patient confidentiality, but it does not alleviate, for me, the fact that I am vulnerable having exposed my inner self in this

A Cheerful Depression

manner. It is irrational to feel this way, after all what can possibly happen. Nothing. I believe most of this caused by the illness and the feeling that they think less of me because of that knowledge they hold. Perhaps I should affirm at this point that I have nothing shameful to hide, I have covered a lot of what they know so far in this book. Not all, but most. We all must have something that we keep to ourselves. I'm afraid you may have to read between the lines and guess what it is that remains unsaid. The distorted thinking causes me to think that all others are familiar with me and my illness. The knowledge that they don't does not lessen the feeling.

To emphasize how this vulnerability has adversely affected me, allow me to recount a story. It was twenty five years ago and the ANC, in South Africa, was still a banned organization. One of my employees, I will call him Moses, was arrested under the Terrorism Act which permitted the Police to hold him for ninety days without charge. He was being held in a prison south of Soweto, Johannesburg. Anyway I was tasked with visiting him on behalf of the company. To reach the prison meant a drive through the heart of Soweto which was, at the time experiencing quite a lot of unrest and the favored method of punishing those who had done wrong, be it cooperating with the police or some other offense, was for them to receive a "Soweto Necklace". This comprised of a tyre filled with petrol being placed around the person and set alight, a gruesome way to die.

The thought that I may have been attacked by the locals never occurred to me, in retrospect a sane man would have considered this very carefully before driving into a township. I visited without incident and have to believe that the purpose of my trips through Soweto was known, to support one of their own, and that the word had been passed not to impede me in my task. In this I think that modern corporations could learn a lot about communication from groups like this.

Remember that, in those days, the mobile phone was a thing of science fiction and most households did not possess a telephone. It could also be argued that my route was standard or that someone followed me to ensure my safety, after all how could anyone pass the word to millions of people in the short time they would have had notice of my intentions. Anyway, I tell you this to demonstrate my own sense of invincibility, that I was not vulnerable to feelings of fear or trepidation.

As a footnote I would like to add that Moses and I became friends. We ran marathons together. He always managed to finish ahead of me. I would drive him home and visit with him and his family, often staying for a meal. He is now highly placed in the Trade Union movement in South Africa. He deserves his success. He has pulled himself up by his own efforts. He is a true gentleman with a lovely family.

It can be argued that some of the above comes from a lack of trust. Now I have the usual suspects who I will never be able to trust. They are the same as the majority of population. Politicians, banks and such. To mistrust those self-serving institutions is normal. However, I find that my levels of trust in my fellow man are at a new low. We are all shaped by our experiences, at work and at home. It is a sad indictment of myself, more than anyone else, that I have slowly developed a cynicism with regard to trusting others to do as they say, to perform a task to the standards I expect. People, being only human, invariably have let me down. This is not so important at work as mistakes, shortcomings can be rectified and the individual can be trained to the required standard. It is when it happens in the personal life that it is harder to reconcile. I would think that we have all been guilty of betraying a confidence or trust placed in us, to some extent. The level of that failure is in the eyes of the person who has been affected. I have always been able to accept most things, giving the person a second chance. There have been occasions when this

A Cheerful Depression

in itself has been a mistake and has cost me dearly. It has to be done. There is good in everyone, sometimes it just needs a bit of prodding to come to the fore.

The mistrust with which I hold everyone, at the moment, is a product of the depression. It is based on the insecurities I imagine. It is a continuation of the pattern of distorted thinking that is so prevalent. Dealing with the mistrust and feelings of vulnerability is not easy. This is where I must hope that, as the process of healing progresses, it will resolve itself. I look on it in the same way as I regarded the night terrors. Those demons which invaded my dreams were imaginary, in the same way as the vulnerability is imaginary. It has been lurking in my sub conscious waiting to escape, to replace a terror that has been confined to the deepest part of my mind and locked away. It is, of course, different for every person, but these demons have been stored away for many years, and I am sure that not everyone will experience them. I certainly hope this to be the case. Whatever demons lurk in the mind I would not wish a visit by them on any person on the planet.

The worst aspect of this lack of trust is the fact that I do not trust myself. I do not trust decisions I make, constantly arguing with myself as to the best course of action. Debating with yourself about the decision is normal; it is healthy to question your motivation. However, this lack of trust extends beyond that, distorted thinking again. Then, after having decided and acted, I worry for ages that I made the right choice. I do not trust myself in the event of something going wrong.

On a more positive note, I have begun to trust Samuel. I have let him read these pages and have been able to take his comments in a positive manner. It has only taken a year for me to get to this stage, which, in itself, is a bit strange, as I have already told him everything about my life and fears. Still it was difficult it was a difficult step to take, a leap of faith, if you like.

The time spent in between sending him this and our meeting was fraught with anxiety as I debated with myself my actions. Sometimes arguing that his comments would only be good in an effort to boost my self esteem and therefore not honest. Did I believe what he told me? Yes and no. Yes in that it was positive, he pointed out the accuracy of my feelings and the actions I am taking to rectify the distorted thinking, stating that my descriptions were vivid. And, no, I do not trust him to be totally honest with me. This is probably very unfair of me, but part of me believes that to be the case.

I do not know for sure if my coping mechanism will kick in and prevent a relapse. Trust in my mind's ability to think straight, to argue against the distorted thought processes and come out on top, is sadly lacking. Everything requires careful examination and thought to ensure that what I am about to do is as a result of the proper, correct, thought process. This can include the simple task of choosing what clothes to wear. Sounds really silly, doesn't it? An aspect of this which is concerning is the necessity to make a snap decision, on the phone, for example. At times like this I can feel myself going into a spin trying to come up with an answer. A return of an anxiety attack, of proportions unknown since the start of all this, is generally a side effect. The self doubt and the re-examination of the facts, and some imagined facts, are looked at time and time again, until something else comes along to take its place.

I also find that I distrust my short term memory and recall. This, I believe, is more a product of the mind racing off on its own tangents. I can find that I will want to do something in the kitchen and, by the time I get there, I have forgotten what it was I wanted to do. I now write things down if I want to remember at a later time. This can extend to simple acts such as sending an e mail; I will put in the address from the address book and then worry, after it has been sent, that I have inserted the correct address. This despite the message sent confirmation. Another one is posting a cheque to pay a bill. I have to check the stubs to make sure I wrote it in the first place, then I worry that I completed the cheque properly. I have now developed a system to ensure that nothing is forgotten and to confirm that something has been completed. However, I don't trust my own system. I check the contents of an envelope, prior to sealing it, at least three times. Some may say this is bordering on Obsessive Compulsive behavior. I don't think this is the case. It is simply the inability to trust myself, my memory. Logic always tells me that I have done it, I can remember doing it, but the doubt remains. I have mentioned this earlier, the effect of catastrophising, always imaging the worst case scenario, and I am sure that I am, to some extent, still allowing myself to do this. I despise this weakness in myself. I fight it daily, I use every technique we have been taught to try and banish these thoughts. I have a feeling that, possibly, I am trying to hard to fight it, to analyze my reactions, over analysis can be as bad as not enough in some instances. It's hard to know what to do sometimes, what the correct balance is, to correct the process.

I have found some people's memory of the past to be amazing. I think of one instance when I was giving a talk to a group of mature students at the local university. Afterwards one of them came up to me and introduced himself as someone who had attended the same primary school as me some forty years previously. I had absolutely no recollection of this person, but he described the various antics and teachers we had. This is not the only time when someone has recognized me from my schooldays and it never ceases to amaze me that these events are so memorable, especially considering I was at the primary school for one and a half years, and the high school for only three years.

I have discussed before the fear of going into crowded places and this lack of trust in myself only serves to compound this irrational behavior. I don't trust myself to act, or react, in an appropriate manner to any given situation. It is all very debilitating and restrictive. I have to believe that I will regain this self-confidence in myself and my abilities. Failure to believe that basic tenet will be tantamount to admitting defeat and consigning myself to self-imposed isolation.

Extract from journal:

In a panic/anxiety all day, really bad in morning on way to shop, then in afternoon during a walk. felt physically ill, chest pains, shortness of breath. Felt really exhausted when I got home, had a bit to eat and tried going to bed early, I was so tired, but only slept for two hours. Got up for three hours and tried again. This time slept for four hours. So conscious and embarrassed about the fumbling trying to pack the groceries. Sure that everyone was watching me.

CHAPTER 9

Something I have found very difficult after the suicide attempt was the living with the fact that I had tried it, as much as with the failure of the attempt. I know forgiving takes many forms, but the act of forgiving yourself appears to be the hardest of them.

I cannot reconcile what I did with my principles and morality. The fact that I saw a priest almost immediately afterwards and made my confession, receiving absolution did not make me feel any better about myself. I know that the concept of confessing one's sins to a priest is strange to a lot of people, however, I like to think the expression - *"confession is good for the soul"* - is relevant, no matter who listens to the unburdening of the woes. The Catholic Church has us making confession to a priest as an intermediary, a representative of God on earth. I suppose the anonymity and confidentiality of the confessional is also a positive influence. The fact that, not only can you think about the things you feel you have done wrong, but also discuss whatever is troubling you, can only be viewed as a good thing. It is, however, I believe, more about the act of contrition than anything else. Only if you are contrite over your actions can you seek forgiveness, in whatever form.

It is a strange thing that we are often able to forgive others for some real or perceived wrong. A colleague at work for a lie, a partner for an indiscretion, and many other things. However, we are our own worst critics and disciplinarians when it comes to forgiving ourselves for some wrong doing. I know I am hard on myself for my failings, my shortcomings. I am prone to going over and over in my mind what I did, blowing it out of all proportion and mentally beating myself up over it.

This has become even worse during the course of this illness.

I have become unable to accept that I am only human and therefore prone to making mistakes. It has now become such a bad habit that it is a daily battle to try and overcome it. This inability to forgive myself, obviously, does not lend itself to any improvement in self esteem. The whole circle of distorted thinking kicks in again and the resulting destructive spiral into low mood and self loathing.

Not only have I found it extremely difficult to forgive myself for the suicide attempt, I have found that events from the past, keep popping into my head. The mistakes made are magnified. Everything is my fault. That *"what if"* scenario I have discussed previously. Logic tells me that yesterday is gone and nothing can be done to change anything. The distorted thinking process, however, tells me different. Many hours can be spent thinking how events could have been changed for the better, merely by a word or action. A complete waste of time. The guilt is great and no matter how hard I try to reconcile the event and remind myself that nothing can change it, if I made a mistake, then I have to forgive myself. After all, the guilt is perceived. There is no reason to feel guilty about the past. Therefore, it should be easy to forgive myself.

I used to have a boss who, if someone made a mistake and was being hard on themselves, used to ask "did anyone die?" Obviously, the answer was always no. However it put the matter into perspective. It could be rectified and was not as serious as we lead ourselves to believe.

I know from the groups I have attended that I am not alone in this. Whilst all of us have done things we may regret, we get over it. Forgiveness is generally always granted in some shape or form. An apology is accepted, provided, of course, that we feel genuinely contrite about our behavior. Others suffering from a depressive illness have made comments which have almost exactly mirrored my own feelings on the subject.

A Cheerful Depression

As they have said, it is easy for someone to offer forgiveness, to say the words. It is completely different for them to be accepted at face value. There is always the lack of trust that what they said was true, that they meant it. You see how all the factors always come back to the same thing – the distorted thinking process. It can be the same if you stand in front of a mirror and address yourself. You can mouth the words, you can mean what you say, but you cannot believe even yourself. There are always the questions. Why am I saying this? Can I possibly mean it? How can I believe the word of someone so full of guilt, who does not trust the workings of his own mind?

Still, no one said it was going to be easy. No one promised a quick fix. At some point the positives will outweigh the negatives and logic will prevail making the need for forgiveness unnecessary. When a realization will dawn that there is nothing to forgive.

In an earlier chapter I mentioned that I believed that Hell was a state in which life was bereft of God. Possibly it is only God who can offer me the forgiveness I seek. But that raises the question, when do I know that I have received God's forgiveness? Some would argue that it is Faith that supplies the answer to that question. If we have faith in a God then surely we must have faith that God is all forgiving. However, in the way as we don't know how EFT works, is it not natural to question something that cannot be explained by the best minds in the world? This is possibly another example of distorted thinking. The doubt in one's own ability to have faith. The need for some tangible feeling, taste, a knowledge that something has happened. I honestly do not know if I am currently in a state which is bereft of God. Nothing that is happening here and now leads me to any conclusion other than He has given up on me. How I rectify that is beyond me. What is the use in praying if there is no feeling that you have achieved something by that prayer? In much the same way as hope, I don't know what I want, what I expect. If there was some kind of feeling which made its way into my mind, some indication in my consciousness that things were changing, would it be a sign from God or would it be that my condition was improving. I know this is a bit deep, philosophical even, but it is one of the questions which plague me daily.

I would like to believe that I have not been deserted by God. After all, through the course of my life I have never received any indication that God is either with me or against me. I have only had my belief to go on, and, now, it just is not enough to sustain me. I am certain that there are theological arguments to explain this loss of faith. I have heard of priests of all denominations who have experienced such a loss of faith. But I have never heard an explanation for them getting it back again.

I know that after my suicide attempt I thought that I had been given a second chance, an opportunity to put things right. What I had to put right I do not know. Maybe it was to write this book and try to help, in some way, others who are suffering from some form of depressive illness. I do find it all very confusing and frustrating. Am I looking for too much? Is this a form of destructive introspection? It may very well be, but if we don't ask these questions of ourselves are we not becoming mindless automatons?

That is the problem with this illness. It has forced me to ask questions of myself. Questions which before, I knew the answers to instinctively. There is nothing in the text books or group discussions which help. I know that if I posed this problem to a priest he would tell me to trust in God and the answers will come. To doubt is normal, Thomas had to stick his fingers in the marks left by the nails on Christ's body before he believed. It truly is very difficult to believe in anything if you don't believe in yourself.

A Cheerful Depression

I am reminded of the trust a small child places in its parents. It is absolute. They have not yet developed the mistrust that comes with having been let down. If their parent tells them everything will be alright and they will ensure that it does, then the child believes it implicitly, and the parent will do everything in his power to make sure that it indeed the case. If only life could be that simple and uncomplicated. To suffer from a loss of faith, not only in God, but in all aspects of life, is, I think, one of the cruelest aspects of this illness.

But it is not only the major issues with which I have difficulty forgiving myself. Everyday tasks and goals which have been not completed, sometimes not even attempted, invoke a tremendous amount of guilt. The perceived recriminations weigh heavily on me and I *"punish"* myself for my failure. This does not entail anything physical. It's all in the mind. I cannot forgive myself my sloth, disinterest or procrastination. This is particularly true with friendships I have ignored, let slip away. I know that it is not because they care about me and want to see me; it is because they care too much. I cannot accept that, I do not want anyone to care too much. It is too much of an inconvenience for me. That sounds terrible but it's true. In one way I want to call them, yet in another way I want to remain on my own. They say that no man is an island, however, I find myself marooned on a very small island, a piece of coral of my own making. I do feel very guilty about this and I hope that, one day, not only will I be able to forgive myself for pushing them away, but that they will find it in their hearts to understand and forgive me. It could be argued that if they don't, then they were never true friends anyway, and I am, therefore, not missing much.

All of this is, of course, distorted thinking and I have to try and turn it around, challenging these thoughts and trying to put a more positive spin on things. Reminding myself that everyone procrastinates on a daily basis, that everyone sometimes need time on their own, to be selfish and indulge themselves. So what I am doing is normal to a certain extent, I am only allowing my mind to blow all things out of proportion. I find that exercise helps to ease the guilt of not having done a particular task. It gives me the feeling that I have accomplished something positive. That I can end the day and tell myself that it has not been a total waste of time. I can rationalize my shortcomings and go to bed in a more positive frame of mind. Of course, there are times when, no matter what I have achieved, I cannot shake my low mood and going to bed in that state generally causes me a poor night's sleep. This is a self perpetuating problem. A bad night's sleep, then tiredness during the day, another poor sleep and the tiredness increases. As this progresses then the mind goes into overdrive as to the reasons, the procrastination becomes greater as the fatigue kicks in, the concern going to bed is that it is going to be another sleepless night.

In these circumstances it requires a great deal of will power to motivate oneself. I use the reasoning that if I exercise, even for a brief period, and use my mind during the day then I will inevitably sleep well. The body's defenses will kick in and ensure a sleep to repair itself. I find this does happen and know, during the days when I am struggling with my thoughts, that, sooner or later, something will click and I will snap out of it. This certainty has taken a few months to evolve. It is only by looking back and remembering previous occasions when my mood has dipped and then recovered can I accept it, make some sense of it and rationalize my behavior.

It could be described as the power of positive thinking. Remember Oddball in "Kelly's Heroes" - *"Think Positive, Man"* – well it can work. Being positive and challenging each and every negative thought is the key to success with this illness.

On the opposing side is the necessity to adopt the habit of congratulating oneself on things accomplished. This is hard in

A Cheerful Depression

the beginning as we have always taken these things for granted, going to the shops, for example. However, it is a positive to have achieved this and I find that the way to remind myself that I have done something good is to literally say it to myself, usually out loud in front of the mirror. It is not easy to adopt this habit. It requires challenging the negativity and forcing yourself to remember what you have done. Remember Samuel and his eternal positive outlook when I first started seeing him. Even on the worst days there is always something which has been done, no matter how minor. To many this may seem somewhat asinine, but remember this distorted thinking ruins self esteem and when that happens it is hard to see any good in yourself. By reminding yourself, recapping, if you like, of the day's events then, with some effort in the beginning, you will always find something positive.

One aspect of this stage of the recovery process, having gone through the courses, is the frustration caused by knowing the reasons for the mood swings and behavior patterns. It is frustrating in that the cause is known, it is part of the recovery process, and the methods to try and challenge this behavior are available to you. However, the sinking into a low mood is remorseless; the feelings of low or zero self esteem are an omnipresent force. I suppose that the fact that there is recognition of this fact is, in itself, progress. The fact that this behavior can be challenged a positive thing. It does not diminish the feeling of helplessness, the ongoing certainty that you are not in control of your own mind and the way it works. This introspection can be harmful as it permits the feeling of failure to come to the fore as strongly as ever. It can feel like no progress has been made and that it is back to square one.

This, of course, is not the case. I have, when this happens, tried to remember what it was like a year ago and make a comparison. Again, this is easier said than done, as it does feel as bad. I have found, however, that I the fact of reminding myself about this am sometimes beneficial in lifting me, if only for a short time. I have found that these mood swings into the depths can vary in length from a day up to a couple of weeks. When they hit I have no motivation, I lack the ability to concentrate and experience no enjoyment in anything I do. Unfortunately, this applies to cricket, which I dearly love to watch. It is indeed a hopeless feeling. Sometimes, I have found that I snap out of it as quickly as I drop into it. When this mood is present I find that it present when I wake up. Then the feeling of hopelessness starts, the feeling that there is nothing worthwhile going on in my life, that there is nothing in the day ahead or in the following days, to look forward to. In this instance it is still difficult to get up and take care of the morning ablutions, eating, exercising and such.

I have mentioned before how I would like someone special in my life. But that cannot be now, not yet anyway. I could not imagine having someone hovering over me, trying to take care of me. I look on the fact that I live alone as a blessing. I have to do things. I have to go to the shop, I have to cook. If there was someone here with me, it is entirely possible that I would abdicate all responsibility for these everyday chores and then sink further into the mire of my mind.

I have, recently experienced such a low. It lasted for almost three weeks. I found that I could do nothing apart from the necessary. I had no interest in anything at all and, importantly, no enjoyment of even the simplest of things. A terrible state of affairs, especially when it coincided with the cricket first test and one-day international against the Kiwis. On several days I went back to bed in the middle of the day. I do not know why I wanted to climb under the duvet, but believe it was the security I sought. I felt very guilty about this and really beat myself up over it. It seemed the vicious downward spiral had me back in its grasp and was not going to relinquish control easily. It really was a waste of three weeks. I performed on automatic. I had to use every ounce of will power to get out of the house.

One thing I found that helped me out was the realization that if I succumbed to these feeling that I was in grave danger of then suffering from acrophobia, and that was the last thing I needed. Attempts to challenge the thought processes were in vain, however, I attempted to do so. My failure to alter my mood was frustrating and annoying, merely adding to my low mood, until I almost gave up allowing myself to let it run its course.

I have often joked, since I found out the definition of bipolar depression, that I would have preferred being bipolar. This means that the individual often experiences very high creative, active spells as well as very low spells. My argument was that if I was bipolar, then my better days would be highly productive, I would need less sleep and could then accomplish much more. Less sleep does not concern me as much as it used to, I have become accustomed, during my low spells, to poor sleep patterns, the difference is that, as I am, I am not at all productive as a result. I generally waste my time sitting around trying to snap myself out of my mood. Of course, the downside is the low mood swings and the lack of creativity they cause. I do not know if bipolar sufferers experience a sense of accomplishment at the highest moments of creativity, but it is certainly something I would like to experience myself. I have not, since the illness started experienced any lasting sense of achievement or satisfaction over anything I have undertaken and completed. It is a fleeting emotion which I enjoy only until my mind combats the feel good factor with arguments that it could not possibly have been as good as I had thought it to be.

As a result of this latest dip I have asked that my meetings with Samuel be increased back to a more frequent, weekly basis. I had wanted desperately to try to go longer periods without any help but it was not working. I reason that trying to cope on my own had a good motive, insofar as I would feel some sense of accomplishment if I did manage. However, I have felt that things have been getting on top of me again. Everything seems an insurmountable mountain to climb. Samuel did remind me that it is easy enough to get hold of someone during moments like this. The only drawback is that I did not want to go out or talk to anyone. It would also have dented my pride that I had to revert back to more frequent meetings. It had, after all, been my suggestion that they been decreased. I am sure, however, that this was the correct decision. It does help to talk things through. It is true that when you talk about feelings they can gain some perspective. There is also the reassurance factor, the fact that such dips such as I have, are normal. Everyone experiences them and they are nothing to worry about.

Another reason that I reinstated the more frequent meetings was due to the fact that I was finding my anxiety levels increasing as the time for the appointment drew closer. The longer I spent between meetings the higher the anxiety levels climbed. It is hard to admit, even to myself, that I am not quite as far down the road to recovery as I would like to think.

Much to my chagrin another thing that does not appear to be improving is my ability to cope with anything that is outside my normal comfort zone. I am sure that there has been progress in this direction, however, most of the time it does not feel like it. For example, if there is to be a visit to the doctor, a phone call that has to be made, and there is time to reflect on it, it seems an impossible task. I believe that some of this is down to the fact that I permit my imagination to run away with me. I start by planning it out, then my mind will wander into the realms of what may happen. It is always the same worst case scenarios that come to mind. This when the particular task may not be threatening in the least, when it is,

A Cheerful Depression

under normal circumstances, something which we would undertake without a second thought. This invariably leads to panic at the thought of doing it, a build up of anxiety until it is completed. Always, without fail, it is not as bad as I had blown it up to be.

There is an initial sense of relief followed by concerns that I had completed it fully. That lack of trust in myself, the sense of self belief that I am capable of doing something properly is disturbing. This in turn leads to anxiety over what I may or may not have forgotten. I have never forgotten anything yet, but the feelings remain for some time afterwards. Logic does not prevail in these circumstances. Challenging the thoughts and replaying the event over and over in my mind does not lessen the feelings. I cope with these feelings by resigning myself to the fact that it is over and done with, anything can be sorted out at a later date. The anxiety felt before and during the event is disproportionate and uncontrollable.

Again the fact that I know what I am doing and what I am feeling is superfluous. The ability to challenge this negative thinking pattern seems to be waste of time, although it obviously is not the case. Further, there is nothing anyone can say to make it feel better. It has to be proven, there has to be an end result which shows that I have coped with the event. Of course, this is not always possible, sometimes there can be no tangible result, and the feeling of not having dealt with it successfully remains for a long time.

On the positive side I find it useful and necessary to actually compliment myself on undertaking a task, whatever the perceived outcome. This I find, as I have already said, is best done in front of the mirror. I have gotten over the fact that it may look stupid. No one is, I hope, ever going to see me doing this.

There are also times when I believe that I am using writing as an excuse for my failure to seek interaction with others. Writing is, by its very nature, a solitary affair. Do I write as an excuse for not going out, for not talking to anyone during the day? Or do I write because I enjoy it and see a result at the end of the day? I would like to believe that I do it because of the latter although I continually question my motives. When I am in the mood and can gather my thoughts, it is indeed a pleasurable experience. More often than not, I question my ability as a writer. I can look at what I have put down and think it to be a lot of drivel. At times like that I think I should give up and delete the whole file. However, something inside stops me doing that. I tell myself that even if no one but I read anything I write it will have been a worthwhile exercise. These arguments with myself, the introspection is challenging the negativity of the depression. The issue of low self esteem is proving to be one the hardest things I have to deal with. I know this to be true of others I have met who suffer from depression.

That is, I believe, another reason for increasing the visits with my key worker. The necessity to remind myself that I am not alone with this type of negative thinking. Reassurance, if you like, that all I am feeling, the low moods and self doubt are normal, are a part of the recovery process. Also the assurance that things are getting better. It is so easy to let myself slip into a downward spiral that I need the discussion to open up to someone and tell them how I am feeling. A lot of the time just talking about it brings the answers I seek. During my discourse I can come up with answers to the questions I am raising. I am sure this is true for everyone. Whenever I was asked at work to offer advice, I found that the best way was to ask questions which made the other person provide their own answers, to make them think for themselves. Quite often what they wanted was reassurance that whatever decision they were going to make was the right one. They only needed a push in the right direction for them to give themselves the answer. So, in a way, I am using that experience on myself. We all have the knowledge and experience to make the correct choice, sometimes, though. It just requires that little bit of help and guidance.

Yet another purpose is the discussing of hopes and ambitions. These can seem unrealistic and unattainable at times. It is difficult, sometimes impossible, to answer a question as to what I want out of, or to do with, my life. I don't know the answer to that, and if I don't the answer myself how can I possibly answer the question. I suppose the one thing I do want, is to be happy again. The bog standard answer which everyone seeks. In my current state, however, I do not know what happiness is, I doubt if I will recognize it when and if it comes along. It is yet another intangible goal. Does money or love make you happy? Will my mind and the negative thoughts take over and refuse to allow me to accept happiness in whatever form it takes. It is a hard question to deal with. I often wonder if the optimism that I sometimes feel is solely the result of a chemically induced state. What would I be like if the medication were to stop? It scares me that I may not be able to cope without the medication. Not that it is addictive in a physical sense, more that it is addictive from a psychological point of view, holding together my mind in some semblance of normality.

If, for example, I was to take a holiday, I worry that I might not be able to cope if something were to go wrong. A lost suitcase, a delayed flight could tip me into an anxiety attack while miles away from my support system. I also ask myself if I would be more conducive to socializing or if I would remain withdrawn. The thought of getting away is, therefore, both appealing and frightening. Again, I know that these thoughts are as a result of the illness and that logic dictates that I would be perfectly alright, but the uncertainty remains. Again in the thinking process of planning some form of break is the catastrophising aspect which comes to the fore. Every time I think of something like a flight, my mind starts producing worst case scenes. What if the plane, train or whatever, crashed? What if I was the subject of a robbery and lost my passport, or money? These thoughts spring unbidden to override any pleasantness the thought may bring. This, of course, is illogical. I have no idea how many miles I have traveled during my life and none of the above has ever happened to me.

Of course, all this inhibits my chances of finding that elusive state we call happiness. If I do not go out of my apartment and look, then there will be no chance to even start the search. In a perverse way, the avoidance issue is a protective mechanism, protecting me from any situation which may be hurtful, in the emotional sense, or from the fear of fear itself. However, as they say with the Lottery, you have to buy a ticket to have any chance of winning. I have found it very easy to make excuses to myself to justify my inaction in this regard. I am perfectly aware of what I am doing and justify that as well. The rationale I use is feasible to me, but when I discuss it I realize how weak and feeble the excuses are, it does not make it any easier to deal with, it merely adds to the sense of failure and low self worth. I do know that the longer I keep avoiding the issue the harder it will eventually be to take control and do something positive. Something else that's easier said than done.

We are our own worst critics. This can be a good thing under normal circumstances. However, it can be destructive if it is permitted to become too overt. To criticize oneself beyond reasonable tolerances drives one to the lowest point possible as far as self esteem goes. I believe that that the introspection and analysis of every thought process can be just as self destructive. There has to be times when the thought process has to be left to run its course, no matter how unpleasant that may be. There has to be an acceptance that it is happening. This is not surrender to the evil within, it is a mild capitulation. It is, at times, best to deal with the issues, or at

A Cheerful Depression

least, run with them, than to fight them, failing and then suffering the recriminations for that failure. They do generally pass as the mind runs off on another tangent. My own way of dealing with this capitulation is to close my eyes and let things develop, using only a small portion of my brain to rationalize the process. At times this can last for twenty minutes, sometimes, over an hour.

It is definitely less tiring than working hard, inducing the anxiety and the muscle tenseness, and can be moderately therapeutic, insofar as the thoughts have run their course and are out in the open. If a herd of cattle stampedes the effort does not go into stopping the run, it goes into turning the herd and letting the run abate naturally. I think it's the same principle with my mind. Let it run, turn it, and it will stop of its own accord.

I have found the above to be particularly true after a meeting with my key worker or a group session. I am always left feeling drained, physically and emotionally, with my mind racing over the content, what was said, how it was said, how I reacted, or didn't react, continuously analyzing and being critical of myself. Often I was too tired to fight the thought process and let it run. I then found it was the best way to deal with it, it always ran out of steam sooner or later. This is only my way of dealing with my thoughts; everyone has developed their own little techniques to use. It's a matter of experimenting and finding what works for you.

CHAPTER 10

I have developed a lot of foibles and idiosyncrasies over the past year. Because I am on my own they do not bother anyone else, I imagine that if I was living with someone, however, they would probably drive them up the wall. Much of the things I have described in this book would be enough to test the patience of a saint, so I suppose that I am fortunate being in this solitary state of grace.

I have already mentioned the behaviors that I am now comfortable with, as comfortable as anyone can be. I like to think that I accept the way I now am, although I would like to change a few things, and will have to wait on this as the recovery process progresses. Small things have assumed an importance far greater than they have ever had. Some would describe some of my behavior as bordering on the Obsessive Compulsive. I have a routine which absolutely has to be followed. A break from this routine is disconcerting and upsetting. The reason for any departure is irrelevant even if I am to blame for any disruption, through oversleeping, for example. I can get quite bad tempered with myself, chastising and berating myself for my laziness or ineptitude. This is particularly bad when my mood sinks to a low for whatever period of time. The longer it lasts the worse I berate myself for not having achieved the goals I set myself. Of course, this is self perpetuating the low mood and the danger of falling into the whirlpool of the downward spiral increases exponentially. As an example, prior to going to bed at night, it is necessary to follow exactly the same routine to ensure the apartment is secure prior to falling asleep. I start in the kitchen checking appliances are switched off, move through the lounge checking plugs there, not just looking but touching to make sure everything is unplugged. Then I check the locks on the front door before going to bed. A failure to do this in the correct sequence results in doubts being raised in my mind

A Cheerful Depression

as I lie in bed and necessitates getting up and going through the whole procedure again. I do not suppose it terribly bad as I only perform this ritual once, but it is something that absolutely has to be done.

It is much the same in the morning. Two cups of coffee immediately on rising followed by the morning ablutions. I require myself to washed and dressed by 07h00. Later than this and the day has started off on the wrong footing. Only once I have fulfilled my requirements and am dressed can I sit and watch the morning news before going out for a walk. You can see now why this could drive someone else to drink!

It has also become necessary for me to set my goals for the day on the previous evening. By doing this I know I can go to bed with everything outstanding to be completed having been incorporated into my schedule, my self-imposed schedule. The morning routine now incorporates these objectives and the time frame I have set myself for completion becomes an imperative. If for some reason one of the goals has to be postponed for any reason I see it as my fault. I should have done it sooner. One example of this was when I dropped a new prescription into the pharmacy. On that day they had one of the medicines but not the other. They offered to let me have the one and then pick up the other the next day. I said I would collect them both at the same time. I accepted this as a minor glitch, although I was less than happy about having to go out again the next day, it didn't fit into my routine! When I returned the next day they told me they had received the missing one but had now run out of the medicine they had the previous day. Outwardly I accepted this but inwardly I was blaming myself, furious that I had not taken the option of just taking the one, then it would be finished. As it happened I had return on two more occasions before my prescription was completely filled.

Quite obviously these events were completely out of my

control, with the exception of taking the one available the first time. However, I punished myself all week for my failure. It is these things which assume an importance way beyond the actual. They are no longer an everyday part of life. They require meticulous planning and, most importantly, they require being 100% completed in the time frame I have imposed.

This is all part my coping mechanism. There are as many of these as there are people suffering from a depressive illness. Each person finds the best way to deal with it, the method they are most comfortable with. I find this routine and the setting of goals on the previous evening permits me to go to bed and sleep with nothing outstanding on my mind. Should there be something I have forgotten or have put off planning, I find that my sleep is disturbed and restless until the matter is resolved. I believe this harks back to the idea that I am pursuing some form of perfection in my daily dealings. It is entirely possible, indeed, likely, that I am holding myself to far too high a standard. Conversely, there are times when procrastination sets in, a sloth for which I loath myself. However, as I try to keep reminding myself, it is necessary to do what I want to do as opposed to doing something because I should be doing it. There are tasks which cannot be put off. Paying the council tax, for example. To delay in something like that only causes more worries and concerns, resulting in restless nights and anxiety. No matter what happens, I always manage to find a way to perform these necessary functions. I may not like it, but it has to be done.

I am now a different person than I was a year ago. I would like to think that I am a better person. I think I am more understanding, more tolerant of others weakness and habits. I cannot see me reverting to the more sociable, outgoing kind of man I was, I cannot see myself in the same job I had previously performed. I have perhaps, more than anything, grown more introvert, have gone back to a time in my

A Cheerful Depression

younger years when self sufficiency and self reliance were the by words. I cannot say whether or not this is a good thing, it does work for me at the moment. Such behavior could possibly be defined as cowardice, because I do not want to face people or situations. Be that as it may, it is how I have learned to cope with my illness. There will, until such time as a full recovery is achieved, always be the feeling that people can read my mind and see the turmoil raging inside. I know this to be utter nonsense, but it does remain a formidable force to be dealt with.

The habit of challenging these and other negative thoughts is now a habit and is something which I do daily, sometimes hourly, in an effort to banish the downward spiral and remain in an positive frame of mind. It is still strange to me that normal, everyday tasks retain such an importance and high degree of thought. The process of recovery in this regard seems to be dragging on forever. I can only hope and believe that this will also be resolved in the course of time. And that is the secret to combating this illness, challenging every thought that pops into your head, which seeks to drag you down. It is not easy, but, hey, who said life was easy? Even when it is a habit which is hardly noticed the process is established.

One of the worst things about having completed the three group therapy sessions is the fact that I now recognize my behavior, the good and the bad. I know when I am slipping into a low mood. I know when I am having an anxiety attack. I know there is nothing life threatening about this. I know the discomfort and pain is a real thing but is not caused by heart problems or anything like that. I can recognize when I am being negative and feeding my own fears. When I am thinking of the worst case scenario. However, even knowing all this does not mean I do not slip into a low mood or anxiety attack. It makes it worse because I now understand what is happening and am still virtually powerless to prevent it.

Here, again, I think I am guilty of trying over analyzing everything that happens to me. I am constantly aware of my thought processes, watching for any sign of weakness. I am so busy doing this that I think I miss out on some of the more pleasurable things that happen. Take a beautiful sunny morning, the gentlest of breezes, sun warm on the face, the roads and streets still bereft of traffic. The only people up and about are those who are walking their dogs before setting off for work. This should be a highly pleasurable experience, especially in Scotland. Why is it not so? I find that my awareness is taken up by the concept of time. The time I have allowed for a walk. Then the fact that my mind is working all the time, not always in a bad way, but this means that I have to concentrate, that in itself being a distraction. The preoccupation of challenging my thoughts has now become almost an obsession in itself, I have now to learn to take time for myself, to sit in the park and enjoy the day. I am looking forward to the day when a book becomes engrossing, when a film is enjoyable as a whole. I truly believe that this is a danger for all of us; we must learn to be selfish, to take time to do what we want to do as an individual, to leave behind the worries and concerns.

How we strike this happy balance is beyond the scope of my knowledge at the moment. Again it is down to each person to find their own way of dealing with it. Perhaps children make the crucial difference, possibly a partner or relations. We must use all the tools at our disposal to achieve this most important of goals.

A huge plus for me at the moment is that the night terrors have stopped. There are still the occasional nightmares, largely unremembered. These are a part of all our lives and differ vastly from the terrors that invaded my dreams and caused long sleepless nights. The unseen malevolent forces may still lurk in the shadows of the darkest recesses of my mind, but they remain there. We all have our phobias and

A Cheerful Depression

fears which surface only occasionally and I am extremely glad that mine have diminished so much. Sleep has become, again, a pleasurable experience, something to be looked forward to and enjoyed. It is good to wake in the morning and feel refreshed. How much of this is down to the medication remains to be seen. I will not allow myself to speculate and then begin to worry about the time when the medication is withdrawn. I have been told that these night terrors were merely a symptom of the whole. I will go through the rest of my life carrying my fear of snakes. After all it is healthy to avoid the infernal creatures at all times anyway. The only advice I can offer with regard to night terrors is to talk them through and persevere. It is a fact of life that nothing lasts forever. It would be physically impossible for the body to sustain that amount of terror and lack of sleep. Its defenses will kick in and prevent any harm. It is definitely horrible at the time and I cannot begin to imagine what it must be like for someone sleeping in the same bed or room. When I was experiencing the worst of them I would often wish that I had someone to hold me, in much the same way as a mother holds a child, and reassure me that it was all just a dream. But then why subject someone else to sleepless nights?

My memories have also begun to resume normal proportions and perspective. Most of the time I can allow memories to surface and relax in the fact that they will not be as traumatic as before. There are still regrets over things I wished I had done differently, things I wish I had said at the time, or actions I could have taken to ensure a different outcome. Hindsight is a marvelous thing; however, what is past is past; no matter how hard we wish we could change it. There are still moments when my mind goes off on a tangent, evoking less pleasant thoughts. I accept this and do not fight it as much as I used to do. It still amazes and surprises me how these memories are so clear and well defined. Whole conversations and sequences of events can be recalled with little or no effort. They can become rather jumbled sometimes as my mind jumps from one subject to another.

Although these leaps may seem random at the time, there is always a thread which can be traced which leads to the conclusion that the mind is operating in a reasonably logical manner. How nice it would be if time travel was not a thing of fiction and we could go back and change things.

I find that now I can remember people with a fondness as opposed to feeling the guilt that pervaded the memories in the past. I can now rationalize the fact that nothing which happened was my fault. There was nothing I could have done to change the outcomes. On the whole this lessening of the guilt is a relief. I would imagine that the feeling is the same as an innocent person charged with a crime would feel when the jury confirmed his innocence. The difference being that I was the judge, jury and executioner rolled into one. It was, I know now, a symptom of the illness that these feelings overwhelmed me. I cannot find it in myself to judge myself less harshly, but now acceptance is easier. With this acceptance comes a certain degree of peace, a quiet that places things in their proper place with the right amount of perspective. I know that for me to say – forgive yourself – sounds easy, trite even, but it is true it is necessary for you to forgive yourself to accept forgiveness from others. My goodness, all that sounds a bit philosophical, but it's true.

While my long-term memory appears to be exceptional, my short-term memory is atrocious. I can stand up to do something in the kitchen and, by the time I covered the short distance I have forgotten what it was I intended to do. I know this is not a symptom of any illness. It is the lack of concentration that still affects me. This condition is dictated by the mind still running at full speed. Ducking and diving from one subject to another in quick succession. It can be frustrating but focusing the mind is the way I have found best to counter this. It's the same as losing the car keys. You

A Cheerful Depression

retrace your steps and movements until you locate them. Should I have a thought, something to do with an idea I have for my writing, I write it down on a notepad I carry. It sounds bad but it isn't a great inconvenience. It is merely a matter of adapting to the current circumstances.

My faith has not been rediscovered as yet and this bothers me to certain extent. I believe we should all have faith in one form or another. I sometimes think that my actions, especially my suicide attempt, will never be forgiven by God. I cannot blindly accept that it is so. I am finding it hard to accept forgiveness at face value, an intangible that I cannot feel, see, taste or hear. Perhaps this is still to come in the future recovery. Or, it is possible that the new me is a tad more cynical than the old me. That, of course, is a contradiction in terms with what I have previously said about maybe being a better, more understanding person. Or is it that I am that person only as far as others are concerned? It looks as if I still have some way to go with the issue of forgiveness.

One thing I do believe is that, had I been younger, I would have entered the priesthood after my suicide attempt. I think I would have made a good priest, even prior to the last year. My life experiences have given me good grounding for dealing with all sorts of problems and now I can add depression to that list. When I think about this I often ask myself if it would be to escape the pressures of the modern world or if it would have been purely with the intention of serving both God and my fellow man. I cannot answer that honestly. However, I can state that to question one's motives is healthy. I know that when I do question my motives now, it is tempered by the thought that they may be moving along as a result of the illness. However, that is a mute point as I am far too old to be accepted into the priesthood.

In conjunction with the above wish is the realization that it may be possible to do something useful with the knowledge and experience I have gained. I have yet to further explore this avenue and have no idea where it may lead me.

One thought I had was to help with the outward bound courses for the Prince's Trust. This, I think, may be more suiting to my skills than sitting in an office, as a counselor, for example. Whatever the choice I make, I would like to think that I may be able to help others overcome some of life's difficulties.

One thing I can be sure of is the fact that I am no longer a passenger on the Titanic waiting for the iceberg to hit and sink into the abyss. I have regained some control over my own life and destiny. I am gradually working my way through the ranks to become captain of my ship. I know, and I have to keep reminding myself, that there is still some way to go, but I am nowhere near the pathetic state I was in a year ago.

Also I know that what happened to me, the depression, is not my fault. It happens, it can happen to anyone, from any walk of life. Yes there were certain things that made my illness a bit more difficult, events which most people, thankfully, do not experience in their day to day living. However, a depressive illness can, and does strike anyone. The stigma attached to it is only in the mind of the individual. Even companies now recognize that depression if a major source of absence through sick leave. I know of some who have qualified people to help employees through their illness, and who have trained Human Resources personnel to recognize the symptoms in their early stages.

I do not know what has happened to the others I met during the course of the three group therapy courses. I hope they are managing to regain some semblance of normality, that their lives are becoming as fulfilling as they once were and that they have again found happiness.

A Cheerful Depression

What can I say about all the people who have helped me through this? Nothing except that they have been absolutely fabulous. They have given of their time and expertise. They have been patient and understanding, diligent and caring. The care provided by the NHS is often bemoaned but they do work very hard. I do know that when I first started on this journey it was with the GP and that he did everything in his power to help me. The referral came through quickly and the support network that was put in place was efficient. It is my fervent hope that no one has to go through the depths of despair that I did, that the help will be provided as quickly as it was for me. It does require the initial effort, the courage to face up to the fact that something isn't right. The recognition that depression is as real as a broken leg and can be treated. It is not something to be ashamed of. It is a real illness and is becoming more common with each passing day.

I do not like the aging process but I will never resort to any artificial means to retain or recapture my youth, with the possible exception of owning a Yamaha 750 motor bike. In today's traffic probably an expensive to kill myself! Here's another quote:

You can't see me, but I'm always around you.
Run as fast as you can, but you'll never escape me.
Fight me with all your strength, but you'll never defeat me.
I kill when I wish, but can never be brought to justice. Who am I?

Old Man Time

That may indeed be the case, we all have to die. It is the last great experience we have. But I will go kicking and screaming. I have already covered the manner in which I would ideally like to die. I do not believe there is any dignity in death. To die with dignity is a myth, in my opinion. All we can do is live with dignity, death in whatever form is not dignified in the least. It is messy and unpleasant. I hope my wishes will be adhered to, particularly if my demise is to be prolonged with the use of medication. I do not want anyone to sit by bedside while I am in a semi conscious state and rambling incoherently. My death will be the same as my life, a very private affair. I refuse to submit to the humiliation of being remembered as a waxen, burbling idiot, with all manner of tubes protruding from the orifices of my body. Not the ease of succumbing to despair, the taking of my own life because there is no tomorrow. I will never again permit myself to go through the agonies of the last year. My pride as far as admitting to being ill will never cloud my judgment and prevent me from asking for help. I have been as low as I ever want to be and I will not permit myself to sink there again.

When I'm back on my feet again, I'll learn to walk to tall again, I'm not going to fall again, I'll learn to be strong. I can think of a few choice words for Old Man Time, but unfortunately they are unprintable!

CHAPTER 11

And that is that. I said at the beginning that I hoped it would be cathartic. Well, it has been, insofar as it has reminded me of the skills given to me during the group therapy sessions. Skills which I use daily to combat the distorted thinking which is still prevalent in and controlling, my life. It has also made me realize how far I have progressed along the road to recovery, although, at times, it certainly does not feel like it. I still have work to do before a full recovery is attained. But one step at a time, always moving forward, gradually overcoming the negativity and bad thoughts. Always battling the *Beast,* sometimes winning skirmishes, sometimes, battles.

Have I become a better person as a result of all this insight into my mind? I would like to think so. One thing is for sure, I am a different person in comparison to two years ago. More compassionate and caring would be my goals, possibly more tolerant and definitely more emotional. Although I haven't cried during *"Neighbors"* recently!

I also said that I hoped that, in some small way, it would be beneficial to others who may recognize themselves in the story. I sincerely hope that has been the case. It would be absolutely marvelous if I have helped someone prevent a repeat of what happened to me, if I have achieved the recognition of symptoms and helped in the process of an early visit to the GP and the proper diagnosis.

In yet another way, I hope that anyone reading this who knows someone suffering from depression will accept that it is an extremely debilitating illness which cannot be cured by *pulling yourself together or having a cup of tea.* That it is a combination of life's events, and a biochemical reaction in the brain. It is an illness which is treatable and from which a recovery is possible, likely. It only takes time and a lot of understanding on the part of those on the outside looking in. Your patience and understanding is important and is greatly appreciated, although it may not be shown at the time. It is easier to talk about a subject to someone who has a grasp of the contents. All you can do is listen and offer comfort when things look bad. I fervently hope that my story has provided an insight into the distorted thinking processes which prevail and are, initially, unstoppable.

When I started this book I had an idea that it might be difficult to recount the events. It has been incredibly hard to revisit the past year. At times I have felt like giving up, it was disturbing for me to think where I had been and remember the feelings and emotions of those times. Am I sorry that I failed in my attempt to kill myself? Over the past year there have been many occasions when that has been the case, when I have come close to trying again, more successfully. Now, however, I have plans, modest and achievable, for the future. The trip to Seville, for example. I can think of the future a few months in advance with some degree of optimism and hope. Possibly I have developed hope in Karma, Destiny or Fate, call it what you will, that things will come together and I will have a life again.

If there is a moral to this story – it must be to recognize that something may be wrong and seek help as soon as possible. It is the same admonishment you hear every day with regard to any illness – early treatment is the answer. Please do not do as I did, it only causes an untold and unnecessary amount of grief for both yourself and those close to you. I feel I have wasted two years of my life and nothing is going to give that back to me, however, I feel I have learned a lot about myself, and that is of some small consolation.

I would also, at this point like to thank, from the bottom of my heart, all those people who have put up with me, listened to me, been patient and who have provided me with the skills

A Cheerful Depression

which now help me cope better with the illness and everyday life. I do not imagine for a minute that I have been the easiest person to deal with. One thing has remained a constant – I am still a stubborn old fool with way too much pride! May that never change.

On a positive note, good things have emerged from this episode of my life. I have learned to play the guitar. Not to the level of Eric Clapton or Jimmy Hendrix, not yet anyway, but on a more modest strumming level, in fact I am so bad that, if I had been a musician on the Titanic, the passengers would have abandoned ship well before it hit the iceberg! I will be conversationally proficient in Spanish, which I hope will be put into practice when I holiday in Seville, later in the year. And, of course, I have written this and two other books. All I have to do now is gather the self esteem and confidence to let someone other than myself, and Samuel, read them, and accepts any comments as constructive.

In all likelihood I will never again have to endure the daily commute to Edinburgh on the 06h33 train, which always leaves at 06h36. To endure the crowded sidewalks, the chattering tourists and the wingeing guests. It is entirely possible that the end of my working life will see me stacking shelves or pushing trolleys in the local supermarket. Who knows? Maybe I will meet that someone special there! Samuel's positive influence still shines through. And that, in itself, is greatly important, be positive and do the best you can. No one can ask for more.

No matter how bad the outlook is, there is hope. There will always be a tomorrow. It may be hard to get through the night, it may seem impossible, but you can do it, with a little help from your friends, however, not Lucy in the Sky with Diamonds, as the Beatles sang. Persevere and things *WILL* come right. There is professional help out there and they are very good at what they do. No, that is an understatement, they are great. They are caring and invaluable in the healing process, guiding us down the path, putting obstacles and setbacks into perspective, allowing us to grow and recognize the best way for ourselves.

I will leave you with a quote, which I use to remind myself of life lessons learned and the fact that time will kill me, not myself.

Time is a great teacher, but,
unfortunately, it kills all its pupils

Louis-Hector Berlioz

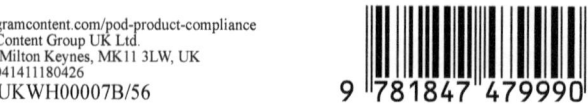